IT **DOESN'T** HAVE TO **HURT** TO WORK
A PATH TO FREEDOM

ERIN J. PARUSZEWSKI

Founder and CEO of Alkalign

BALBOA.PRESS
A DIVISION OF HAY HOUSE

Balboa Press books may be ordered through booksellers or by contacting:

Balboa Press
A Division of Hay House
1663 Liberty Drive
Bloomington, IN 47403
www.balboapress.com
844-682-1282

Interior Image Credit: Erin J. Paruszewski

Print information available on the last page.

ISBN: 978-1-9822-7582-2 (sc)
ISBN: 978-1-9822-7584-6 (hc)
ISBN: 978-1-9822-7583-9 (e)

Balboa Press rev. date: 11/05/2021

CONTENTS

For my girls, Ava and Elle. You inspire me every day to be a better human. Seeing the world through your eyes has opened up my own. May you always love yourselves as much as I love you.

AUTHOR'S NOTE

This book is not meant to wow you with facts and figures about how 36 minutes of exercise and three daily servings of kale will increase your happiness and longevity. It's meant to tell you that exercise and food don't have to be painful or joyless and to give you permission to stop following the latest fitness and food fads. I wrote this book to inspire you to think about your health in a holistic way and to encourage you to start tuning into your body and your intuition. I'm challenging you to stop punishing yourself and start prioritizing yourself. It's time to ask: *What kind of exercise and nutrition does* my *body actually need?* My book is backed by research and learning. But more importantly, it's based on real-world experience. I personally found freedom when I realized my body and belly didn't have to hurt to work. Through my fitness studios, I have helped thousands of others do the same with a functional approach to life. This approach is about real bodies in their natural habitat doing everyday movement. It's about real people evolving into better versions of themselves.

My goal is not to tell you exactly what to do and how to do it. No one but *you* can tell yourself the best way to eat or exercise for your particular body. That's because self-care is an inside job. My goal is to educate, inspire, and empower you with a back-to-basics approach to living a healthy life and with my own story of transformation—how I went from falling apart physically to finding alignment in the ways I move and nourish my body every day. At the end of each chapter, I'll challenge you to pause and reflect on how what you've just read applies to you. Taking time to slow down and look inward is a fundamental, and sometimes uncomfortable, part of evolving as a human. Thank you for trusting me with your time and energy as we embark together on the journey of understanding why functional movement matters.

It really doesn't have to hurt to work.

INTRODUCTION:
SEARCHING FOR THE SECRET TO A HEALTHY LIFE

Here's the question I hear all of us asking:

What is the secret to a healthier and more vibrant life?

Here's my answer:

Eat better. Move better. Sleep better. Connect better. Feel better.

It sounds simple, right? But real life has a knack for getting in the way. Work, kids, pets, soccer games, family obligations, vacations, and pure, unadulterated exhaustion wreak havoc on our health goals. We can barely find time to swing through the drive-through for a quick snack or coffee on our way to work or in between evening carpool pick-ups, let alone incorporate a consistent, nutritious food plan *and* move our bodies on a regular basis. And who has time for a full night's sleep? Let's face it. Our health is the first thing we take for granted and the last thing we think about after we've turned in a big project or tucked the kids into bed at night.

Prioritizing ourselves and our well-being has gone by the wayside. I bet if I asked you to name your top priorities for this week right now you'd easily rattle off a quick list, but exercising daily or making sure all of your meals contained whole foods is probably not going to make the list. That's because we brush off the notion of taking good care of ourselves right now. Instead, we say we'll do it "when we have time later." But later turns into tomorrow or next week or next month, and, before we know it, we're flipping the calendar to a new year. As a result of not prioritizing ourselves and our overall well-being, we are experiencing more physical and mental illness than ever before.[1,2] I don't have to convince you—you're living it.

To make matters worse, there is so much conflicting information in the world about what it means to be "healthy." When we reach for answers on how to live a healthy and vibrant life, we're overwhelmed by thousands of options, hundreds of promises, and millions of gimmicks. We are constantly inundated with fast fixes and the latest fads, all promising we can lose weight and feel great with less effort. But poor eating habits, processed foods, and fitness fads are making us feel worse, not better. And unfortunately, the health and fitness industry is all about the quick and easy sale when it comes to its bottom line. I know this firsthand. Finance and the healthcare industry used to be my day job. It's frustrating but eye opening to realize we live in a culture where "healthy" is defined not by ourselves, but by money-driven marketing messages that prey on our deepest insecurities. Rarely do we stop to question if the defining source of what's "healthy" is a trusted voice or proven method. Instead, we blindly believe the promise of stronger, faster, better, skinnier "in just 10 days," and when it doesn't work, we blame ourselves for falling off the health and wellness wagon and seek out the next short-term solution. Sound familiar?

It sounded familiar for me, too, until I realized that health and wellness are a *lifestyle*, not a pill you can swallow or a movement you can consolidate into seven minutes. The truth is a fast, magical solution to food and fitness simply doesn't exist (if someone tells you it does, *they're lying*). This may sound depressing or hopeless because we all want the quickest and easiest path from point A to point B in order to maximize the time we have to do the things we love. But I know from experience that "fast" fitness and fat-free food were my fast track to injury and illness. On the flip side, mindful movement and whole food are what my body craves. Understanding this reality was actually quite liberating for me, and I think it will be for you, too. Because without the distraction of the "latest and greatest" or "the next best thing," we find time, energy, and better focus to commit to smaller, incremental changes that allow us to feel better consistently over time. This is what I mean when I say health and wellness are a *lifestyle*.

But I didn't experience this lifestyle transformation with the snap of a finger. It took some work at first. Like most of us, I was used to living my life on autopilot. One event or goal led to the next, and my fast fitness and fad diets were along for the ride. I always wanted to look good for my upcoming vacation, family gathering, or class reunion, so every time I was on the verge of a big event, I would suffer through the self-inflicted punishment of increasing the exercise and decreasing the calories. I wanted to *look good*, even at the expense of *feeling good*. I honestly thought it *had* to hurt to work. But that kind of mindset was only punishing my body, not prioritizing it. As a result, I showed up at far too many sandy beaches and social settings with a body that looked seemingly "healthy" on the outside but felt nutritionally deprived and physically exhausted on the inside. For me, setting aside the assumption that exercise and eating well are only for a point-in-time purpose has been liberating and has resulted in feeling better physically and emotionally. Believe it or not, it has been easier and more rewarding to maintain a healthy lifestyle that's relatively consistent day to day and involves incremental habit changes than it was to endure the physical and psychological whiplash that accompanies the food and fitness fads.

For most of us, pursuing this kind of healthy lifestyle requires a massive shift in our mindset—a mindset that's deeply ingrained from years of practice, influence from our family of origin, and input from our culture and society. Shifting our mindset to accept and implement sustainable change is challenging, especially when it flies in the face of everything we have believed to be true up until this point. Transformative change isn't easy, but it's possible. That's why you're here with me. Because I've learned that the secret to transformation is training for life over the long term, not just training for one moment in time. That means being a student of your own body, taking a holistic approach to food and fitness, and making time to rest, reset, and connect with yourself and others, which leads to a healthier, more vibrant you over time.

So if you want to find your path to transformative change, then this book about why functional movement and holistic nutrition matter is for you. Let's get started.

FUNCTIONAL FUNDAMENTALS:
DEFINING THE TERMS

A Functional Approach to life is a holistic practice that incorporates a balance of all the health pillars needed to live healthfully: whole-food nutrition, mindful movement, sleep, hydration, and human connection.

Functional Nutrition is about eating to nourish your body on the inside versus eating to look a certain way on the outside. This way of thinking prioritizes fueling your body with whole unprocessed foods to optimize your health so you can be the best version of yourself.

Functional Movement describes the different patterns your body makes during the day. Functional movement allows you to accomplish daily life tasks. The seven functional movements are: walk/gait, rotate, lunge, push, pull, squat, and hinge.

squat   rotate   hinge   pull/push   lunge   walk/run (gait)

Functional Fitness is the focused and intentional practice of functional movement to improve strength, alignment, balance, and stability in order to enhance your performance in your everyday life, doing everyday activities. Instead of working out just to work out and burn calories, the purpose of functional fitness is to exercise in a way that will improve strength; proprioception, or the brain's understanding of where the body is in space; and mobility, or the body's ability to move freely and easily.

PRINCIPLE ONE:
BE OPEN

"A mind is like a parachute. It doesn't work if it is not open."

Frank Zappa

wasn't always into a functional way of life. In fact, if someone had predicted when I was in my 20s that I'd stop long-distance running and do an about-face on my exercise philosophy by the time I was in my early 30s, I wouldn't have believed them. If someone told me that I would significantly improve my life with the practice of basic functional movements and things such as myofascial rolling, a self-massage technique to improve mobility and reduce pain, I would have rolled my eyes and completely disregarded it. *Who's got time for stuff like that anyway?* My reality check came when I was told I would need a hip replacement unless I chose to make a change in the way I was exercising and taking care of my body. I was 24 years young. And it still took me six more years to make the necessary changes to my fitness mindset.

Pushing my body to exercise extremes was my jam up until that point. It was what I knew best and how I got the fastest results. It was also how I stayed moderately thin while still binging on beer, bagels, and all the candy I could consume. As a former ballet dancer and serious athlete (at least, I took myself seriously), I was a hardcore, type-A, extra-double-stuffed Virgo who ran seven marathons and participated in more triathlons than I can remember over the span of a few short years in my early 20s. It was how I stayed sane from long days in a corporate office. Back then, I thought stretching was a waste of time and "tapering," or running less, as race day approached was for the weak. Strength training wasn't even a consideration. As a result, I had lots of injuries, including a torn ACL, shin splints, hip issues, shoulder issues, and painful plantar fasciitis. Yet I forged on. I wasn't going to let any of that "nonsense" slow me down. I was raised to be tough and wasn't going to quit under any circumstances.

As you can probably already tell, I had a fixed mindset about a lot of things. And if I dig a little deeper, I also felt like I had to earn things. From the calories I consumed to my parents' approval, I always felt like I had to work for everything. I ran to earn my beer and candy, to be able to eat whatever I wanted without gaining weight. I was good at running and loved to earn the happy hormones and infamous "runner's high." I tracked my mileage, my caloric burn, and my heart rate from every run in a spreadsheet. I was putting in the work and had the data to prove it! I also earned titles for my list of life accomplishments, for example "Boston Marathon Qualifier" and "Boston Marathon Finisher" *twice*. Running was a big part of my identity. It was who I was and what I would always do. That is, until I started having more aches and pains. As those aches and pains slowed me down significantly over time, I started realizing I didn't enjoy running as much as I used to, and it didn't make me feel as great as it once did. The torn ACL and hip replacement warning should have been the final straw, but they were actually the first signs I noticed that something wasn't right. You could say I was in a bit of denial up until those injuries. Running filled a void in my life, and I wasn't prepared to let go of it or what it represented. Looking back now, I can see I was spending tons of time and money at various body workers to address my injuries, and training for races started making me extra cranky. But I was too busy living my life to notice—training for the next race, and the next one, and so on. Despite the hip replacement warning from my physical therapist, I continued to run consistently until the age of 31. It was like a 911 emergency wake-up call was on the line, and I put it on hold. For six years.

Eventually, I started running less and engaging in other types of workouts, namely spin and barre fitness, two fitness fads that hit the West Coast in the early 2000s. I joined a gym, regularly went to group classes, and began exploring movement in a different way. And before I knew it, I wasn't running at all. The very thing that was my *everything* was now *nothing,* and I was OK. I was actually better than OK. I looked better. And by better, I mean I looked stronger and healthier. But most importantly, I *felt* better. Ironically, as I stopped pushing my body to its limits with long runs on the open road, I started making giant leaps forward in other areas of my life.

It would still be a few more years until I found what I now refer to as a more functional approach to life, but I was feeling better and beginning to see life beyond the intense workouts and rigid spreadsheets I updated daily. Life changed in other ways, too. I met my husband, Tony. We got married and moved to Menlo Park, a suburb of San Francisco, where I continued climbing the corporate ladder. As I rounded the corner into my 30s, life looked good on the outside but still felt incomplete on the inside.

I was in a senior role at work and making decent money, but something was still missing. No longer in denial about the way I was mistreating my body, I felt better thanks to my new workouts. Feeling better physically gave me the mental space I didn't know I needed to dream about life beyond my corporate cubicle. It was actually those workouts that would eventually be my ticket off the corporate train.

But I'd have to face those demons of my denial again, alongside those punishing practices I thought I had set aside.

WE ALL HAVE ISSUES

Every summer as a kid, my parents would take me to see the New York City Ballet perform at the Saratoga Performing Arts Center where I grew up in Upstate New York. Those performance nights were this girl's dream come true as an aspiring dancer. In fact, my mom's goddaughter Catherine was in the ballet, and once I was lucky enough to get a sneak peak behind the curtain with her. She brought me backstage to meet the dancers and collect autographs. But I was shocked by how many dancers were standing outside the backstage door smoking cigarettes. It was a confusing sight for my adolescent eyes. There stood those beautiful, graceful ballet dancers whose profession depended on their athletic capabilities, and they were *smoking cigarettes*. Didn't they know smoking was bad for them? And didn't they know there were hundreds of little girls and boys in the audience who looked up to them? Smoking was not the role-model kind of behavior I expected from these professional athletes. But little did I know back then that smoking curbed their appetite and very few of those beautiful, graceful dancers fueled their bodies properly on any level. It was their way of staying super thin. At the ripe old age of 10, I remember feeling a twinge of judgement directed toward those dancers. How could they? And yet, years later, I would struggle with destructive patterns of trying to control my appearance.

If I'm being honest—and I am, because honesty, transparency, and authenticity are important to me—I have battled with all sorts of demons in my lifetime, from body issues and obsessive exercising to diets and disordered eating. My guess is most of you can relate on some level, too. We all have our struggles. Even though I've come a long way, I still wrestle with some deeply rooted beliefs about fitness and food that are hard to shake. While on paper I have always appeared to be happy, healthy, and balanced, this picture of perfection wasn't always my reality. Spoiler alert: what we post on social media or how we portray ourselves to the outside world isn't often an accurate depiction of what's happening on the inside. What started for me as the quest to be skinny morphed into a fear of food, thanks to my super-sensitive insides. And for a while, I teetered on the brink of *orthorexia*, an eating disorder that involves an unhealthy obsession with healthy eating. Unlike other eating disorders, orthorexia mostly revolves around food quality, not quantity. This was convenient because starving myself was never one of my strengths. But I thought if I could control every single ingredient that went into my body, I could avoid embarrassing bathroom-related blunders, too. As with all things *extreme*, this mindset was neither sustainable nor was it the example I eventually wanted to set for my daughters, Ava and Elle.

Sharing my story with you is hard—it feels a bit too raw at times, and I don't like admitting my denial or my fears to a broad audience—but my hope in sharing my story is that you will feel the freedom to be open and honest about your story, too. Being open and honest with yourself is the *first step* to a better you. It's also the best way to be *human*.

REAL, RAW, AND HUMAN

One of the most helpful ways we can be open and honest with ourselves is to be real about our fears. You've probably heard this suggestion: "be curious, not judgemental." When we get curious about our fears, we see they are what hold us back from being a better version of ourselves and from living life to its fullest potential.

I vividly remember one of my earliest fears in life: drowning. And I remember exactly how that fear started. My younger brother, Andrew, was 3 years old when he almost drowned in a relative's swimming pool. I was 4 at the time. The pool was custom built and made of dark stone.

There was no bright-blue-plastic liner on the bottom or number signs to mark the depth. Andrew and I were playing on the steps during a family reunion when he lost his footing and disappeared under the water faster than I could blink. I was completely helpless, as any 4-year-old would be. Luckily, Uncle Jack spotted Andrew and jumped in the pool to save his life. Andrew was safe and sound wrapped in a towel in my mom's arms after those harrowing seconds, but I had nightmares for years and an ongoing dread of drowning. In my adolescent and teen years, I could technically "swim" thanks to the swimming lessons my parents invested in at our local pool, but that didn't matter. I was always nervous in the water. And a few washing-machine-like tumbles in waves at the Jersey Shore didn't help, either.

When I moved to San Francisco after college to begin my career in investment banking, I was already running marathons, so I jumped on the triathlon train, too. Cycling became a close second to running as I embraced the opportunities for even more calorie-burning cardio sessions. If duathlons were a thing, I would have loved them even more— sans the swimming element. But, unfortunately, in order to participate in a triathlon, my land-loving self was going to have to get comfortable swimming in open water.

My first triathlon was on Catalina Island in Southern California. I nervously anticipated the start. I had invested in a wetsuit, which I finally figured out zipped in the back and not in the front as I originally thought. This was rookie mistake No. 1. I had also trained in a pool and not in open water. Rookie mistake No. 2. On the day of the race, I ran toward the ocean, dived into the waves, and immediately had a panic attack. I remember how cold and salty the water was and how it was hard to catch my breath as my head bobbed above water. There were hundreds of people thrashing their limbs all around in the water as they literally tried to swim over me. And my heart was racing like it did all those nights when I woke up with the same bad dream—the one where Andrew was drowning again, but this time he was drowning at the end of a pier in the ocean, and everyone at the party on the beach was too busy to notice.

Still stuck in the middle of a swell of triathlon participants on their way around the swim course in the waters off Catalina Island, I popped my head up like a gopher, frantically searching for the nearest lifeboat. I desperately wanted to quit, but in a split second, I realized I had never been a quitter and wasn't going to start then. I took a deep breath, found the courage to start moving my arms again, and doggy-paddled out to the buoy. I looped my arms around it and stopped for a few seconds to tread water. Then I rolled over onto my back, still gasping for air, and back-stroked for my life *all the way around the course.* If memory serves me, it was a ¼-mile swim, but it might as well have been 100 miles that day. I made it back to shore and was never more grateful. For some, this experience might have suggested an end to competing in triathlons. Not me. I just kept upping the ante.

Two years later, I was still on the triathlon circuit in and around San Francisco. I had left banking and had more time to enjoy both the competition and the camaraderie of my newfound tribe. I hadn't drowned yet and decided the ultimate opportunity to face my fear was to sign up for the Alcatraz Triathlon. I was a history major in college and had been obsessed with Alcatraz ever since we visited the national historic landmark on a family vacation when I was a kid. Like most people, I wanted to know if the prisoners who escaped Alcatraz actually made it out alive or perished in the frigid, shark-infested waters. If so, would I, too, succumb to the same fate as I attempted this latest deranged Darwinian stunt?

To get ready for the triathlon, I spent months training in the murky, dirty waters of Aquatic Park. The prep alone was almost more than my sludge-phobic self could handle, but I trudged on. My sister and I were committed to finishing the triathlon together. My mom and aunt even flew out to California from the East Coast to cheer us on. When race morning arrived, we bravely boarded the ferry out to Alcatraz Island. But this time we didn't disembark at the visitor center. Instead, we jumped off the side of a boat into the same shark-infested waters in which three prisoners had risked their lives for freedom. We were many years beyond their infamous escape, but I felt a strange sense of solidarity with them as I jumped into the water that morning. I remember literally shaking from head to toe while I stood waiting to jump. Right after I nervously peed in my wetsuit, I gave myself a little pep talk. *You're not a prisoner of Alcatraz, but you have been a prisoner of your own fears. If you make it back to shore in one piece, you'll conquer those once and for all.* And I did. It wasn't pretty. In fact, I think I probably had one of the slowest swim times of any participant thanks to the unique and inefficient combo of dog-paddle, freestyle, and backstroke, but I did it. I conquered my fear of drowning that day.

But there were deeper fears left unconquered, namely my fear of getting "fat" if I ever let up on my extreme fitness regime.

My Challenge to You: So let's get real for a moment. *When was the last time you were open and honest with yourself about your fears and your denial?* Are there things that come to mind for you as you read my story? If so, grab a journal and a pen, or the notes app on your phone, and jot down the fears and areas of denial that pop up for you. There is no need to do anything with them right now. Naming them is half the battle.

KEEP DIGGING

"Maybe you are searching among the branches, for what only lies in the roots."

Rumi

Hindsight is always 20/20. I would have made a lot of different choices over my lifetime if I had known then what I know now. And I'm certain the same is true for you, too, because I hear it from the friends, colleagues, and clients who walk in and out of my fitness studio doors every day. There are regrets and realizations including "I wish I had stayed out of the sun," "I wish I hadn't gone back to that boot camp where I hurt my back," and "I wish I had prioritized my health earlier." But, alas, we can't go back in time. We hopped on the metaphorical treadmill in our young-adult days, and we just kept increasing the speed, at all costs, without a glance over our shoulder at the other options around us. This was me with running, and it's you with whatever is driving you to keep pushing your mind and your body to the extreme.

Now that I'm beyond those days of activities that accelerate wear and tear to my joints, prioritizing a preventative and functional approach over the fleeting feeling of a runner's high seems obvious to me. I'd choose safe movement and methodical exercise practices any day over the latest flashy fitness fad. *But why doesn't this resonate with everyone, and why do we all keep running back to bad habits and broken bodies?* This is the question I've been trying to answer for many years and what I continue to explore in my life's work. We all have a human tendency to gravitate toward the promise of the perfect body or the perfect life without considering both the short- and long-term implications of our behaviors. It's the reason why people we know listen to "fitness gurus" who make them get in a bathing suit so said "experts" can circle their cellulite and point out their problem areas (yes, this *actually* happens). Why would we even allow that kind of message to infiltrate our brains? Because we're hooked on the promise of a better body more than we are on the promise of a better life. We care more about the outside than we do the inside.

When we really think about it, we can all agree that daily activities like walking, breathing, sitting, standing, writing, bathing, and wiping are all essential. Yes, I said *wiping.* And if we were to lose our ability to do any of these things, our lives would become significantly more challenging and less pleasant. However, human nature is reactive. It's the "squeaky wheel gets the grease" phenomenon. So as long as things in our lives, including our bodies, are in relatively decent working order, we don't think about how important basic activities are to our daily lives. Or, like many of us in severe denial, we don't think about them unless our bodies or our lives are broken beyond repair. *Even then,* it can be hard to get past the ingrained beliefs and ongoing obstacles that seem to stand in our way. It's safe to say we generally take things in life for granted until they are broken. That's why it's no surprise that it's hard to get most of us to care about practical and useful ways of moving our bodies beyond the bright and shiny studio lights or the facade of Instagram filters. Functional isn't perceived to be fun. Functional isn't believed to be sexy. However, last time I checked, having someone wipe your backside because you're too injured to do it yourself isn't very sexy either. But I digress (no pun intended).

Back to the ballet dancers I saw smoking cigarettes at the backstage door. Skinny trumped healthy at all costs for those individuals. They knew how to be healthy, so why did they turn to cigarettes to curb their appetites? For the same reasons football players ignore or conceal signs of a concussion and get out on the field despite the risk of long-term brain damage. For the same reasons professional athletes pop pills so they can keep performing through the pain instead of heeding the warning signs their bodies are desperately trying to give them. For the same reasons you and I torture ourselves with grueling workouts and starvation diets. We convince ourselves that more is more when it comes to exercise and less is more when it comes to food. And we compare ourselves to everyone around us.

ROOTS THAT RUN DEEP

What I've learned through both research and experience is that these reasons come from roots that run deep for most of us. And those deep roots represent beliefs that were sowed as little seeds long, long ago in our lives. These beliefs that have been nurtured by our family of origin and our community upbringing, fertilized by some education along the way, and then fed by influences of friends, family, media, fads, and false promises. We all have these roots, and what we believe to be true about fitness, nutrition, and overall health is both eminently ingrained and profoundly personal. As I reflect back on where I am and how I got here, I recognize a lot of little influences that have shaped my beliefs throughout life. Some influences and situations were positive. Many were not. And a few were downright humiliating. We're not here to point fingers, place blame on anyone, make excuses, or elicit sympathy. In fact, I believe digging down to uncover deeply held beliefs requires an immense amount of gratitude for each life experience we've had and for every person who has shaped us into the individuals we've become. This kind of gratitude includes the good, the bad, and the oh-so messy. Struggles from our formative years and setbacks from our everyday lives are our most profound teachers in life, and they're what propel us on to greatness.

But we have to dig deep to uncover those long-held beliefs that keep us in unhealthy holding patterns—like my running past the pain and pushing my body to the extreme so I could burn the right amount of calories in order to keep eating whatever I wanted—if we're ever going to release ourselves from those beliefs and patterns. You might have heard the phrase "name it to tame it," coined by psychiatrist Dr. Dan Siegel.[3] We have to name our beliefs and tame the unhealthy mindsets that hold us back if we are really going to be open and honest with ourselves. My personal mantra for this is: *live present. be forward.* This mantra is so important to me and the way I run my business today that you'll find it in big bold letters on the studio walls. Live Present. Be Forward. It's the best way to live, and we will get into this in more depth a little later in the book.

BELIEF BLAST FROM THE PAST

Here are some of the mindsets and beliefs that ran deep for me until I recognized them for the lies they were:

Size matters. I grew up in a house and a time when skinny was good and fat was bad. Whether in reference to people or the products they consumed, it was clear that skinny was celebrated and fat was shamed. And I'm guilty of that shaming, too. I still regret mercilessly teasing my younger brother when he went through an awkward adolescent pudgy phase. I called him "fat boy" for nearly a year. I'm not proud of it, but that was the norm back then. No wonder these words are such triggers for me. The only mention of *fat* and *skinny* in my house these days is in reference to avocados, nuts, belts, and margaritas. I also recognize the difference between skinny and healthy. I know plenty of people who look skinny but are actually quite unwell.

Shape matters. I self-identified as "pear shaped" in third grade. *Pear shaped.* Where did I even get that language? Perhaps I picked it up at home. Maybe I heard it from the older girls in ballet where body image and eating disorders were omnipresent. Either way, at age 9 I was already self-conscious about my body and wore an oversized T-shirt over my leotard. I dreamed about being tall and lean like the other girls I looked up to, including a few who were dangerously anorexic. It probably didn't help that my dance teacher occasionally poked the side of my butt and told me to tighten it. Her intentions were harmless, but those pokes are likely the reason I still consider this part of my body a "problem" area. This story is also the reason I was not sad or disappointed when my own kids never took an interest in dance. There was too much pressure to *look* and *be* a certain way.

Bendy is best. In second grade, my dance teacher cared more about the recitals and the sparkly costumes than the art of ballet. She insisted I do "the splits" in all 3 directions before moving up in level. Even back then, my hips were tight. Being the achievement-oriented person I was, I went home and practiced over and over and over. I could wedge myself into a split with the left leg forward, but the right leg and straddle splits were impossible. I felt ashamed, like I wasn't enough. The good news is I knew I didn't belong there, and my mom switched me to a ballet school that was much more accepting of individuals' differences. The bad news is society's universal celebration of flexibility, what I later learned was mostly hypermobility, haunted me for decades. I wasn't the girl who could touch her toes in gym class or could contort her body into some crazy pretzel position in yoga. Being "bendy" was cool. Being tight was not. So I did what we all do when we aren't good at something. I avoided stretching like the plague, convincing myself it was a waste of time. Little did I know at the time that I was dodging a major bullet as hypermobility is a serious condition that leads to a lot of issues later in life. My self-esteem may have been shot, but at least my joints were not. While I now know that stretching and mobility work are key to a well-balanced body, I do feel somewhat vindicated. If that dance teacher were still alive, I would certainly love to educate her on the physical risks of putting hypermobility on a pedestal and the psychological impact of placing an impressionable young girl's self-esteem on the back burner.

Running is the only way to stay thin. My sister, Carey, who is five and a half years older than me and the one I looked up to the most growing up, started running in junior high because she had "never seen a fat runner." I'm certain she was only repeating something once said to her. I'm sure it didn't help either of us that my dad would often tell friends and strangers alike that Carey could play for the Green Bay Packers because she ate so quickly. What teen girl wants to be compared to a football player? So, naturally, I followed in her footsteps and took up running, too. Running was the means to an end for us, and the end was burning enough calories to share an entire Betty Crocker strawberry layer cake, complete with pink vanilla frosting and rainbow sprinkles. This is how I continued to justify my cardio obsession, which later expanded to include cycling and swimming. My innards could be a wreck, and I could feel like crap. But I believed that an unending aerobic effort equaled staying thin and that in the absence of running, I would be fat. One unhealthy belief led to the next, and I felt trapped in a circular reference of shame.

Appearance is always a comparison. To this day, there's a small plaque hanging at the top of the only full-length mirror in my childhood home that reads, "Dear Lord, if you can't make me skinny, please make my friends fat." Need I say more?

Competition is everything. I tried out for the field hockey team in seventh grade and got cut. So I decided to take up cross country because there were no cuts. A girl can only handle so much rejection at that age. But doing one sport wasn't enough for my competitive spirit, so I skied on my high-school alpine ski team until I tore my ACL. I was 15. I had surgery, healed, and went right back to running. I didn't run just to run; I ran to compete and win. Competition and comparison go hand in hand when you're constantly measuring yourself against everyone else.

You are what you do. For most of my life, I've measured my value against my constant productivity and output. And that bar of expectations was set high in my family long before I was born. I used to believe that if I wasn't sweating, I wasn't working hard enough or at all. I used to believe that if I wasn't burning 1,000 calories a minute, a workout wasn't worth it. If I didn't run for at least 45 minutes, it wasn't worth the effort it would take to shower. If I didn't work out two times a day, I was failing in some capacity. I used to believe that if every workout wasn't meticulously documented, it didn't count. And I definitely believed that where there was pain, there was always gain—as long as it wasn't weight gain.

Fat-free is the only option. I came of age at the height of the "fat-free" era of the '80s and '90s. And I grew up in a house where my mom was always on a diet. She did Weight Watchers, counted every calorie, and wore her lightest silk pants to her weekly weigh-ins. Looking back now, I can only imagine the pressure she must have felt and the deep-seated beliefs she must have struggled with on a daily basis for all of this to be so consuming for her. For years, I watched her weigh herself methodically and eat from a small plate using a tiny fork, likely a tip she picked up along the way regarding portion control. She counted calories, so that's what I did, too. None of us ever paid attention to the actual ingredients we were consuming in our fat-free food—the amount of sugar or processed chemicals or overall lack of nutritional value never even crossed our minds. We simply knew that fat was bad and skinny was good. I often joke about how much smarter I would have been had I fed my brain the fat it so desperately needed during my developmental years. And those deep-rooted beliefs at the time applied to both the food I consumed and the body I believed would result. Fast forward to my life now, and this is a concept so incredibly foreign to my daughters. We now know "good fats" nourish and energize our bodies and our brains so we can live life to the fullest regardless of how society tries to label and shame our bodies.

Sugar is an acceptable addiction. My love of sugar came from associating it with the end of every meal as well as every celebration and special occasion. I remember sitting around the dinner table and wanting to finish first so I could claim the coveted "clean plate club" title that evening. We literally had a little teddy bear, a gift from my Avon lady Aunt Cynthia, that had a groove in its butt so it could sit on the edge of the plate. It held a blue heart that said "I'm special," and the bear was awarded to the first kid to finish dinner. It's no wonder we all hoovered our food like Green Bay Packers. Clean plate club meant we could have dessert. I never wanted to miss out on the assortment of cookies, brownies, and other sweet treats my mom baked on a daily basis. During the summer months, we took frequent trips to the local ice cream shop. I was also the kind of kid who spent a lot of time and energy hoarding my Halloween loot, making it last for months so I could retreat to my room and reward myself with something sweet. As kids, the only time we were allowed to have soda was for celebrations and special occasions: birthdays, graduations, holidays, good report cards, and so on. I also remember the great lengths my siblings and I would go to in order to sneak it from the basement fridge when my mom wasn't looking. My brother Andrew and I would prop each other up to grab the Coke from the top shelf and then chug it straight from the two-liter bottle. I also remember obsessively searching all the teacups in our dining room for the antique key that would unlock the cupboard of chocolate chips my mom used for baking. Every year my parents went on a one-week cruise without us. As a treat, they bought us one box of Lucky Charms for the four of us to share while they were gone. That box didn't stand a chance of lasting past the first day. Nine times out of ten, it was ravenously consumed before my parents were down the driveway. My addiction to sugar fueled my addiction to running because I believed that the more I ran, the more ice cream I could eat without gaining weight. I never for a moment considered how all that sugar was damaging my insides and compromising my microbiome.

My Challenge To You: If you want to stop punishing yourself and pushing your body to work even though it hurts, you have to acknowledge the roots of your deeply held beliefs. I shared a few of the rooted beliefs and mindsets that kept me sunk in the same unhealthy patterns for years, and now it's your turn. *What beliefs have shaped the way you take care of yourself with fitness and food?* Grab your journal and a pen, or the notes app on your phone, and jot down the deeply rooted beliefs that pop up for you. Naming those beliefs is how you move out of the denial that keeps you stuck where you are. You picked up this book for a reason, and if you want to move forward and get to the place where it doesn't have to hurt to work, you have to keep digging.

PRINCIPLE THREE:

LISTEN WHEN YOUR BODY IS WHISPERING

"Our wisdom does not just come from what we learn. It also comes from what we unlearn."

Cleo Wade

n 2000, I graduated from Georgetown University with a degree in History and a minor in Spanish. *Hablo un poquito.* My natural inclination as a history major was, and still is, to look back in order to learn from the past. This is how I acquire information about the present and determine what steps I want to take as I move forward into the future. What *was* helps me better understand what *is*. And more importantly, the past gives me a better idea of what *could be*. Combine that perspective with an extreme thirst for the "why" when it comes to health and wellness, and I'm constantly trying to ask the right questions, pay attention to the most helpful things, and make educated decisions with the information I have. This is also why medical professionals collect health histories from their patients. They hope that there is some relevant information about the past that will help better explain current issues and predict future outcomes.

Speaking of the past, aside from one soul-sucking job at Banc of America Securities where I literally never saw the light of day, my post-college life was good in California. I worked hard in various roles and spent my limited free time training for one race after another. But some gut issues that had begun in high school kept surfacing. I spent much of my teens and 20s with debilitating abdominal pain. The only position where I could experience temporary relief was doubled-over with my elbow jabbed into my right side. This was great for my professional confidence. *Please excuse me while I crouch in the corner of the board room doubled over in pain. It will pass as long as I crouch down and apply constant pressure for a few long minutes.* Being a history aficionado, I affectionately referred to this awkward move as "The Napoleon," not due to my short stature but because the French military leader was often photographed with his hand inserted into his coat at his abdomen. He is believed to have died of gastric cancer that had ulcerated and ruptured his stomach. *Good times.*

DEEP IN DENIAL

My gut issues began in high school around the age of 15, the same year I tore my ACL while skiing. I often felt as if I were "bruised on the inside" and so bloated I wished someone could have popped me with a pin. Not to mention the emergency bathroom runs that accompanied the pain. So I did what any health-conscious teenager would do in the '90s. I doubled-down on a diet of fat-free caramel rice cakes and yogurt and an occasional apple (yay, real food!) for lunch. For dinner, my mom usually made some kind of chicken or pasta. She was no Martha Stewart in the kitchen, but I give her a ton of credit for always preparing a hot meal served around the family dinner table. She incentivized us to eat said meal with promises of her ooey gooey, super-sweet and delicious desserts because what she lacked in cooking, she more than made up for in baking (more fuel for my acceptable sugar addiction). Back then, there was no talk about nutrition or stress management, lactose intolerance, or Celiac disease. In fact, in my family, we didn't talk much about anything labeled "personal" or "private," such as the gut issues I was experiencing.

The summer between my junior and senior year of high school, I was invited to Cape Cod with two families I babysat for on a regular basis. My job was to be an extra set of eyes at the beach by day for four young boys and be the only eyes at night while the parents went out. I had never been to the Cape before and had never been invited anywhere, for that matter, so, naturally, I was thrilled for the opportunity to "get out of Dodge" and get paid. And the best part was that the two families rented a big white house on a cul-de-sac within walking distance from the beach.

One afternoon, the boys and I were playing in the sand along the ocean. I was sporting my favorite purple one-piece bathing suit with the colorful flowered straps. I loved that suit. Normally, I felt great in it. Except for that particular day, nothing felt normal or great. Something was not right with my gut. It was gurgling and churning—a feeling I was used to from years of being gassy, bloated, and generally uncomfortable. I tried to ignore it because I had a job to do. I was in charge of those kids and determined not to let the parents down. So I continued to run buckets of water from the ocean to the spot in the sand where they were busy building castles and moats. Minutes passed as the gurgling and churning in my gut grew worse. I tried to ignore it, but despite my best attempts, I couldn't overcome the agitation occurring in my innards. In the blink of an eye, the situation went from urgent to emergent. I HAD TO GO. Literally.

Panicked, I signaled to the one parent who was fortunately on the beach at the time. It was a nonverbal signal—a quick wave of my arms that meant *I'll be right back*. Writhing and wincing, I clenched my butt cheeks in discomfort and started for the house. This was happening. Oh shit. OH SHIT! I scurried up the closest sand dune as fast as I could and sprinted toward the house, which was on the far side of the cul-de-sac. There was a wooded path in the center of the cul-de-sac circle. I bee-lined through the sandy shortcut toward the house. I was so close but knew I wasn't going to make it. I just couldn't squeeze my sphincter anymore. So I squatted right there in the bushes, but I couldn't get the flowered straps off fast enough. Like a volcano erupting with molten hot magma, my body was exploding with piping-hot poo. It was an out-of-body experience, and, in that moment, I wanted to be anywhere else but there. Anywhere else but in my body, in those bushes, on this Earth. There I was squatting and uncontrollably pooping in my swimsuit. I was absolutely mortified. I was determined to bury any acknowledgement of that incident as deeply as I buried the excrement in the sand that day.

From that day forward, I bought two-piece bathing suits because they were easier to get off in a pinch. I also started paying closer attention to my gut health, or lack thereof. *Why was this happening? What were the contributing factors?* I started paying attention to what made my belly rumble and why. I don't know why I waited so long. Did I think someone would magically notice I was uncomfortable and fix the issue for me? But denial was easier than the hard work it took to find a solution, so I stayed quiet about the emergency bathroom runs a little while longer. It was an awful existence shrouded in shame.

Eventually, it got so bad that I had a battery of tests: an upper GI scope, a lower GI scope, a test for parasites, a barium enema, and so on. You name it, I had it. All of the tests were negative and inconclusive. Eventually, I ended up in the hospital for exploratory surgery, and the doctors removed my appendix, which appeared "shriveled." They labeled my condition "chronic appendicitis," but I wasn't convinced, especially since the pain continued. Through all of that, not one doctor asked me about what I was eating—which was a lot of dairy and carbs those days. After all, skim milk and bagels were FAT FREE!

Years after the infamous Cape Crap incident (my affectionate term for what was actually the Cape Cod incident), I was confronted with another gut emergency. I went on a double date with my roommate and our respective boyfriends in Washington, D.C. We made a rare trek off campus to see *Shakespeare in Love*. I dressed in my double-date best, which in true '90s fashion included pleated khaki pants, a white tank top, a button-down flannel, a brown braided belt, and, of course, matching brown Doc Martens. The theater was dark, and the love story on the screen mesmerized the audience into a moment of silence. I was captivated—not by the sonnets, but rather by the sound of my own stomach. The feeling was all too familiar. Bubbling. Brewing. Sloshing. And soon to be squirting.

I think I sat deep in denial at first, hoping by some miracle I would not live another fecal fiasco that night. But once again, I waited too long. When the emergency moment arrived, I jumped from my seat and bolted to the bathroom. Pushing open the bathroom door, I simultaneously and frantically untucked my shirt, unfurled my braided belt, and unbuttoned my pants. My fingers were working as fast as possible. The fury of fine motor skills fired as I attempted to unzip and sit. Simple enough. I was sooooo close. But as the old saying goes, "close only counts in horseshoes and hand grenades." Before I knew what was happening, my gut grenade ignited, and it took out everything in its path. *Oh no. Oh yes.* On a date. In the bathroom. At the movie theater. I pooped my pants, *again*. So much for Shakepeare's iambic pentameter or the post-motion-picture make-out session. I triaged the situation the best I could. I cleaned every affected area of my body with all the available toilet paper, ditched my underwear in the trash, tied my flannel around my waist, went back to sit in my seat, and waited for the night—and nightmare—to end.

That episode should have been no surprise considering my college diet. Lucky Charms with skim milk, bagels, pizza without the cheese (because of course cheese has fat in it), more pasta, and beer. It's no wonder I was doubled over in pain with a bloated belly and had to hang Bounce dryer sheets in my room in an attempt to mask the toxic gases that emanated from my body. While I knew enough to know my roommate's Diet Mountain Dew and Slim Fast addiction was unhealthy, I didn't know enough to cut back on Dr Pepper or to consume an occasional cruciferous vegetable at my end. I was still too deep in denial to make different choices.

FUNCTION OVER FASHION

After that night at the movie theater, I immediately adopted some new rules. In addition to "no one-piece bathing suits," now it was also "no belts." I was confident that addressing these surface-level stumbling blocks would help me avoid another epic elimination malfunction. However, I failed to realize that the *symptom was not the source*. It wasn't fashion's fault. It wasn't even my slow response time to the gut gurgling. My issues were indicative of a much bigger source of dysfunction happening in my body. But in the meantime, the safest choice was function over fashion.

Although it wouldn't come to fruition for many years, this was the beginning of uncovering the root cause behind these explosive events so they would never be repeated. It would take years to uncover, understand, accept, and adapt accordingly. But the process completely shifted the trajectory of my life.

DIFFERENT SEASON, SAME STORY

With my embarrassing emergencies behind me, my post-college move to San Francisco initiated the adulting adventure. I worked long hours in banking and didn't have much time or extra money to leave the office for lunch. I kept a jar of fat-free Skippy peanut butter in my desk drawer along with a stash of spoons for whenever I wanted a snack. Breakfast was sugar-laden cinnamon raisin oatmeal. Lunch was a soy-infused veggie burger on a frozen onion bagel with a side of Jolly Green Giant canned corn niblets topped with leftover parmesan and chili pepper from the previous night's pizza. Yup. The nutrition of a 20-something champion. And I wondered why I still felt terrible. But I justified my eating habits, and my denial, with the calories counted and miles logged on my spreadsheets. My output was still greater than my intake, even if my food choices were crap.

The abdominal pain continued as did a mounting number of other issues, such as aches and pains in my hips, knees, shins, feet, and shoulders. My physical body was breaking down at the tender age of 25. I had already seen a plethora of doctors, body workers, and specialists in different fields. Believe it or not, *no one* asked me about my nutrition. No one suggested I stop running or start cross-training. No one inquired about my stress levels. No one looked at the big picture.

Very slowly and over a long period of time, I wised up on my own. I read an article here and learned a new tip there. Then I went to see a kinesiologist I found on the Internet. The first visit was $500 out of pocket, a hefty investment when I was still finding my way out of school loans, but I was desperate. In a consultation, the kinesiologist explained to me that flour and water were acting like glue in my digestive system. She did some physical adjustments to my ileocecal valve, a sphincter muscle situated at the junction of the end of the small intestine and the colon, or the first portion of the large intestine. Its function is to allow digested food materials to pass from the small intestine into the large intestine. The adjustment felt great. She also advised me to "stop eating white food" for two weeks before my follow-up appointment. All I knew was white food. My identity as a cardio queen depended on carbs. I tried for a few days but failed because I didn't know what to eat instead. Sweet potatoes and quinoa were not part of my vernacular, and the lack of education I received on the topic was a big issue because of my lifestyle at the time. How would I train for a marathon without "carbs"?

I fueled myself for a 14-mile run that following Saturday with egg whites, dry canned tuna, and mixed greens. On Sunday, I rode 40 miles through the town of Woodside and literally collapsed on the side of the road in a pile of horse manure. My friend Charles had to bike all the way to his car, two towns over, and come back to pick me up. We went to Buck's, a Silicon Valley landmark, for breakfast afterward, and I lay in the booth unable to move. Yet I refused to eat anything other than egg whites. I continued to feel so awful that I eventually went back to eating the way I normally did. I couldn't sacrifice my job or training for this silly health practitioner who clearly didn't know what she was talking about. I never went back to see her.

KNOWING BETTER, DOING BETTER

Even though being doubled over in pain all the time was horrible and the pain was having a negative impact on my day-to-day living, it wasn't enough motivation to make a change. This way of eating was ingrained in my brain, just like running was deeply ingrained in my body no matter how badly it hurt. I ate all the processed carbs and ran all the miles even though I knew this was not good for me. There was a symbiotic relationship between the two. That was the power of my denial—of my deeply rooted belief system.

Eventually, I realized the kinesiologist was probably right. She was right about the over-processed carbs, but her approach lacked the education I needed to inspire any sort of change in my lifestyle. Instead, seeds were planted slowly over time, and, at first, I bulldozed those seeds with doubt, destruction, and denial. But, eventually, I started making small changes to my diet. For example, I swapped out high-fructose-corn-syrup-infused fat-free peanut butter for the natural kind, which simply contained peanuts and salt. This set me on a trajectory for better food choices overall. After a few more tests and several self-directed elimination diets, I had to face my biggest fear. Dairy and gluten were my top-two sensitivities, which was problematic when I was all about bagels, pasta, fat-free yogurt, and skim milk. Around this time, I also started taking group fitness classes rather than always running alone.

Over time, these little changes made a big difference. And it shifted my mindset regarding fitness and nutrition as something I "got to do" rather than something I "had to do." I didn't *have* to give up gluten—I *wanted* to give it up because it made me feel better. I didn't *have* to give up running—I *wanted* to because finding other ways to move my body made me feel better, too. With each passing year, I felt better. I had fewer flare ups of my GI system, fewer aches and pains, and far more energy and confidence. Smarter eating and exercise meant I felt stronger and more vibrant on the inside and looked better and more radiant on the outside. The truth about what was best for me and my body was starting to sink in, and I was starting to transform. In the process, I learned that no one was there to reward me for making better choices regarding fitness and nutrition, and on the flipside, no one was going to scold me if I didn't. My proverbial punishment was self-inflicted, and my reward was self-realized. And the same is true for you as you transform, too.

My Challenge to You: When something hurts, whether it's a repetitive injury, a recurring gastrointestinal issue, or something else, listen to your body and look at your health history holistically. Then you can start to know better. It's like I tell my kids all the time, "Listen when mommy is whispering, not when she's yelling." By the time I'm yelling (yes, I yell sometimes; remember, this a judgment-free zone), the issue has escalated, and it's a lot harder to reverse course. It's much easier to address a situation in the whispering phase. But listening to our bodies when they're whispering requires change, and change requires action. In the absence of action, history will repeat itself, or it will get worse. So take a few moments to pause right now. Grab your journal and your pen again or the notes app on your phone, and ask yourself, *What has my body been trying to say to me lately? What stands out about my health history? What has my body been trying to say to me all these years?* It likely isn't as obvious, and hopefully not as embarrassing, as the examples I experienced. It could be something much more subtle like mid-day fatigue, brain fog, a dull headache, stiff joints, mood swings, food cravings, or that need for the daily 5 p.m. drink. For now, just notice. Eventually, you will want to take action. But don't rush it. First, just pay attention. And trust your gut. You will know when it's the right time to take the next step.

GET BACK TO THE BASICS

"Take care of your body. It's the
only place you have to live."

Jim Rohn

By now you get the picture that I was great with setting fitness and nutrition goals, but I was terrible at listening to my body until it was on the verge of not working anymore. Once I started listening to my body, I knew what I needed to do, but I didn't always like doing it. I knew I needed to nourish my body with more whole-food nutrition and strengthen my muscles with more mindful exercise. But sometimes I rebelled and binged on things I knew my body didn't like. A few times, I even purged in an act of instant regret. Both options felt terrible. I ate crappy food and went back to my fat-free, sugar-filled fixes. Or I'd tighten up my laces for a long weekend run, even though I was already in a lot of pain. But neither option worked for me anymore. I had to figure out how to be consistent with a new way of *living* and a better way of *being*. That search is what led me back to the basics of functional fitness, which like most people, I originally thought were too "boring" and too "simple" in a world of flashy fitness fads. That is until I realized how much functional fitness was overlooked and undervalued. In reality, going back to the basics in a thoughtful and meaningful way was exactly what I needed to build a stronger foundation for my future.

THE STUDIO STARTUP

It was the spring of 2008 when I realized I was completely unfulfilled working in my corporate gig. On paper, I was helping people, but I felt like a cog in the wheel working at a behavioral health company where I had no idea if the products I was developing were delivering any value to the consumer. I had become an instructor in several of those group fitness classes I was taking, and I realized that teaching classes at 6 a.m. before work or at 7 p.m. on the way home was the best part of my day. That's when I knew it was time to harness my passion and turn it into a profession. There was no denying I had inherited an entrepreneurial spirit from my dad, who started his own business manufacturing screen printing equipment the same year I was born. I was very newly married at the time, and Tony and I were thinking about next steps. He woke up one morning in our San Francisco condo and proclaimed, "I want a lawn to mow." I told him, "I'd like to open a fitness studio." I had been teaching at a barre studio in San Francisco, and there were franchising opportunities available. Tony is a thoughtful, calculated risk-taker, so naturally he responded by saying, "You're absolutely crazy!" I understood his concerns, but I couldn't shake the sixth sense I had that this was my next step. In fact, one of the mantras I live by is, *"Always trust your gut. It knows what your head hasn't figured out yet."* And this was one of those instances. Much like the lag I experienced between knowing better and doing better with food and fitness, my gut was saying go, but my head still had some catching up to do. Through a lot of conversations, we decided it was important for me to do something I loved as well as something that would give me the flexibility to raise a family. We relocated to Menlo Park, a suburb just south of San Francisco we chose for the sunshine and the schools. In 2009, I resigned from my corporate job on the day of President Obama's inauguration. Still fired up from his "Yes We Can" campaign, it seemed like a fitting time to take a leap and make a change that would hopefully effect change in other people's lives, too.

TRUST YOUR GUT

Let's pause for a quick moment and talk about what it means to trust your gut. I don't just want to keep throwing that phrase around without giving it some kind of definition. We often talk about "trusting your gut" or "using your brain." But saying it that way makes it sound binary—like one is better than the other, like it's either/or. But it's a both/and statement because your gut is essentially your second brain. According to Stanford microbiologists Drs. Justin and Erica Sonnenburg, a primal connection exists between the gut and the brain. As they explain in their book, *The Good Gut*: "Our brain and gut are connected by an extensive network of neurons and a highway of chemicals and hormones that constantly provide feedback about how hungry we are, whether or not we're experiencing stress, or if we've ingested a disease-causing microbe. This information superhighway is called the brain–gut axis, and it provides constant updates on the state of affairs at your two ends."[4] Thus, listening to and trusting your gut is of the utmost importance. It's the same thing as using your brain.

FINDING MY WAY TO FUNCTIONAL

I opened my first barre studio in Menlo Park in March 2009, and a few months later, in January 2010, we opened one in the neighboring town of Los Altos. Barre workouts consisted of exercises inspired by ballet. Thus it was a natural fit for me to be a barre instructor, and now a barre studio owner, with my background in dance. I was fulfilling my childhood dream of ballet-like movement everyday, even if it wasn't in pointe shoes with a pink tutu. Barre workouts combined ballet with yoga and pilates exercises, which were in stark contrast to my super-speedy and sweaty cardio sessions but surprisingly effective. I especially craved the slower pace and opportunity to continue exercising without the excessive impact while I was pregnant. I gave birth to my oldest daughter, Ava, two months after we opened the second studio.

In more ways than one, my path to a functional approach to life happened by chance, not by choice. It wasn't something I was looking for, but it was something that had to happen. I couldn't spend any more time living in a dysfunctional body. Even though I had reduced the amount I was running by the time I became a group fitness instructor, classes didn't necessarily feel like "enough." Old habits are hard to break, and I just couldn't stop, even when I knew I needed to. Looking back now, I can see what a gift it was to find out I was pregnant in the middle of launching two barre studios. It felt like the "accidental circumstance" I needed in order to come up with an alternative to running. I also got really serious about my nutrition during that time, inspired by the tiny human I was incubating. My focus completely shifted from how food choices made me look on the outside to how food choices impacted the baby on the inside.

Like so many of us who give birth to tiny humans or new dreams and ideas, I learned and evolved so much in the years after Ava was born. Not only did I want to figure out my gut issues for myself, but I also wanted to fuel my family in the best way possible versus slipping back into what was familiar. I had come a long way in my understanding of the human body and the acceptance of my own body. I knew being skinny was not synonymous with being healthy. In fact, there were, and still are, plenty of skinny people in my life struggling with diseases of the body, such as cancer, and diseases of the brain, such as eating disorders, stress, anxiety, ADHD, and a whole host of other issues. Those issues might have contributed to weight loss, but they come with a plethora of other problems, too. It hit me that in the absence of a strong body and balanced mind, skinny can look pretty scary. So I no longer strived to be skinny because I wanted to be physically and mentally healthy and strong.

Despite these significant shifts in lifestyle and massive leaps forward in mindset, I was still caught off guard by unstable gut health that would upend everything. On one vacation, I ordered a salad without croutons. When the salad arrived with croutons, I simply removed them rather than sending it back. I spent the next 18 hours in pain on the couch in the fetal position with a toddler running circles around me. Frustrated, I went back to the drawing board and endured a whole litany of tests and procedures, this time 20 years after my first round of tests and on the opposite coast. Again, not one doctor asked about my nutrition, even in sprout-eating, avocado-consuming California. I decided to take charge and search for real answers. I did a few more tests to rule out Celiac disease. Thankfully, neither the endoscopy nor the colonoscopy results showed I had the disease despite having the gene. But my sensitivities to dairy and gluten were confirmed with continued trial and error. A bad hip, two fitness studios, an energetic toddler, an unsettled stomach, less time to run, and a lot of fear were the perfect storm for a lot of stress, which only made my health issues worse. It was also the storm that paved the path for me to find my way to better fitness and nutrition and, overall, a functional approach to life. And it all started when I found functional fitness.

So what is functional fitness anyway? Although it is somewhat debatable who coined the term *functional fitness*, the idea of functional training was introduced by a Swedish physiology professor named Per-Olof Åstrand.[5] Functional fitness is the practice of exercise movement required in your daily life to improve strength, alignment, and stability. Instead of working out just to work out, you're working out to enhance your performance in your everyday life doing everyday activities. Those activities and goals depend on the person. For one person, they can be getting out of bed and walking to the bathroom without pain. For another, they're driving the golf ball farther with more power and with less back pain. Functional movement happens every day. Functional fitness is the packaging of those movements into a workout that is holistic, balanced, and applicable to life.

According to the Mayo Clinic: "Functional fitness exercises train your muscles to work together and prepare them for daily tasks by simulating common movements you might do at home, at work, or in sports. While using various muscles in the upper and lower body at the same time, functional fitness exercises also emphasize core stability."[6] Essentially, functional fitness is informed by seven movements: ***squatting, rotating, hinging, pulling, pushing, lunging,*** and ***walking.***

In technical terms, functional fitness is based on real-world situational biomechanics involving multi-planar, multi-joint movements. It's a whole body, holistic, and wholly challenging way to move. When your brain and body do these movements well, you have better posture, better performance, better coordination, better mind–body connection, and fewer aches, pains, and injuries. As I tell my clients, functional fitness is all the rewards of physical maintenance without the risk of excessive wear and tear on the body. A true win-win.

Sounds great, doesn't it? Now that you know the definition and the benefits, you can close the book and head out in search of a functional fitness workout that will allow you to reap all the aforementioned benefits ASAP. But chances are you won't. *Why not?* The challenge with functional fitness as a category is that, by definition, this kind of fitness is "designed to be practical and useful, rather than attractive,"[7] aka functional. In the world of fast and sexy fitness fads, "practical and useful" is not typically what we look for in a workout. We want something attractive. We want the latest fad. The issue with fads, of course, is that they are fleeting. They serve a purpose for a period of time and then expire, like the seasonal pop-up store at your local mall. But your body is here to stay, and how you take care of it matters. Unfortunately, a holistic approach to fitness and nutrition is in direct conflict with the marketing schemes of most companies. No matter how much they pretend to care about the health and wellness of the consumer, money is always the top motivator. In fact, industries such as fashion, food, and fitness thrive off of short-lived flashy fads. See Shake Weights, Snackwell's, Sweatin' to the Oldies, mullets, ThighMasters, and the Master Cleanse.

BEYOND THE BULLSHIT

As a studio owner, I started taking better care of my body in the areas of fitness and food, but once I did, I realized I needed to take better care of myself mentally and emotionally, too. Running a business and caring for a young family is no joke. To be frank, owning a franchise can be hard; it definitely had big ups and downs for me. Taking care of someone else's business is a great way to go as long as there is alignment between you and the leadership of the company. But when there's misalignment, the reality can be really challenging. Because of my type-A, driven nature, I just worked through the issues. It took a painful situation for me to recognize the obvious fracture between the company I thought I was a part of and the company I wanted it to be. That fracture occurred over *a miscarriage*.

I woke up on November 1, 2012, with what I initially thought was a slight sugar hangover. This didn't surprise me because it was the morning after another epic Halloween in our neighborhood. Ava was two, and we dressed her as my sister's beloved chocolate lab, Wrigley. Tony was Dog the Bounty Hunter, and I was a hot dog with a "bun in the oven" because I was expecting again. Together, we were a pack of dogs. (This is how I make myself laugh, friends.) I got out of bed and sleepily stumbled into the bathroom only to discover I was bleeding. A lot. The pang in my heart radiated to my belly and back. I knew it wasn't good. I was due in downtown San Francisco later that afternoon for a studio owners' retreat with my parent company. Long story short, I called the owner of the company and told her I wasn't able to make the retreat because I was pretty sure I was in the middle of a miscarriage. She replied, "Oh Erin, can I tell you something?" "Um, sure," I mumbled. "The same thing happened to a friend of mine, and she really wanted that baby. She was glad it happened." I politely told her I knew the miscarriage was a sign this baby wasn't meant to be but I was going through a lot physically and emotionally at that moment. I wasn't going to make the cocktail hour or opening remarks that evening but would be there the next day. She responded with, "Well, there's never a good time to miss our retreat, but if you're just going to be the girl crying in the corner, maybe it's best you don't come."

Needless to say, I lost more than my baby that day. I lost all respect for the person, the brand, and the business that I had spent four years and all of our life savings building. And to some degree, I lost some faith in humanity. But I gained so much more. I gained clarity, conviction, and another opportunity to trust my gut. Because what I didn't know in that moment was that the loss of one life would completely change the trajectory of another, *mine*. From that day forward, I knew I had to make a move beyond the barre and all the bullshit that came with an extrinsically focused brand. But it would take another two years before I knew what to do. In the meantime, I gave birth to a second beautiful baby girl and named her Elle.

By 2014, I was at a serious crossroads. I was five years into running the two barre fitness studios, and, financially, things were going well. But my mindset had started to shift after that retreat weekend conversation. It didn't help that at every company gathering, the same leader would be inebriated and smoking cigarettes outside the bar, a behavior that boomeranged me to the backstage doors watching the ballet dancers smoke. To say there was a misalignment in values is a gross understatement. Also, I was a different person. When I first opened the businesses, I was a 30-year-old newlywed with a fairly myopic mindset about food and fitness. Five years later, I had discovered more of a functional way of fitness and nutrition, and I had two daughters who I was now responsible for raising. Something needed to change. I could no longer deny the unsettled feeling I had been ignoring for years. I had to trust my gut.

At the suggestion of a close and trusted friend, I hired a business coach, Coach Mary, to help me figure out why I felt like I was constantly living under a black cloud. In theory, I should have been happy. I had a thriving business, a loving family, an amazing community, and my health.

What else could I want? In reality, I felt like I was living a lie. I spent my days selling someone else's ideology, which was not in line with my ethics or morals. I was doing my best to fake it, but it was eating me up on the inside. Even worse, the inner turmoil was increasingly more transparent every time I walked into the studios. I was stressed, cranky, and resentful.

It took a few weeks of discussions with Coach Mary for her to point out that I was struggling because I craved authenticity. I wanted to live, work, and connect in a way that was true to me. I wanted to stand for something that I believed in. I wanted to be a person that my kids could be proud of. I wanted to model a way of living that would inspire them to be good to themselves. More than anything, I wanted them to love themselves. No matter what. But before I could model this for them, I had to believe it myself. After several more months of coaching, my current business, Alkalign, was born.

A BETTER ME, A BETTER YOU

Although I can say with 100% certainty that functional training— the combination of functional fitness and functional nutrition—has transformed my life, I admit there was a 0% chance I would have ever believed in it before I was ready. Timing is as important as mindset. In my 20s, I knew one way—punishing my body by calories in, calories out and eating copious amounts of pasta—and that was, in my opinion, the *only* way. I'm not sure if my mindset was influenced by my yet-to-be-formed prefrontal cortex, my determined and sometimes stubborn personality, or my overwhelming desire to look a certain way, but the combination resulted in a cardio chick who wouldn't quit. I firmly believed in "stronger, faster, better" and "more is more" when it came to exercise. And I constantly battled the messages such as "nothing tastes as good as skinny feels" and "a moment on the lips, a lifetime on the hips" that seemed to be everywhere. Anyone else? It took becoming extremely broken mentally and physically to realize that extremes are never sustainable and are almost always detrimental to our long-term health.

I understand how hard it is to accept something that you don't understand and have never experienced. It's like my lack of enthusiasm for *Game of Thrones*. I've never watched a single episode, so when the rest of the world geeks out about every detail of the finale, I tune out. I have limited capacity for conversation about the latest fad if it's not relevant to me at the moment. But functional fitness isn't a fad. For me, it has become a way of life. And I think it has the potential to become a way of life for you, too. You are reading this book because something about it piqued your interest. A small seed has been planted. How you nourish it is up to you.

My Challenge to You: If you want your body to last, you have to invest in it. All of it. You have to learn to see exercise as self-care and movement as a functional way of life. But the functional way of life requires active participation (unlike a pedicure or a massage—two self-care things you can literally sleep through). Intentional exercise and healthy nutrition require active participation of both our brains and our bodies. They are practices that require us to take responsibility for ourselves and our own well-being, which is why we tend to avoid them. We'd rather be held accountable by someone or something else so we have someone or something else to blame when we derail. But, tag, *you're IT*. Grab that journal or your notes app again, and jot down your answer to this question: *What are you doing to be a better version of you? How are you moving your body in intentional ways and making whole-food choices tailored to your specific needs?* Bonus: *Make a list of the seven functional movements, and write down the last time you performed each one.*

PRINCIPLE FIVE:
LIVE PRESENT.
BE FORWARD.

"You create a good future by creating a good present."

Ekhart Tolle

We have a saying in our home and in my fitness studios: *Live Present. Be Forward.* It captures the mission that drives the business I started to go beyond the barre and is the motto that inspires our lives. That motto is what led me here to you.

Remember how I told you things began to change after I saw the kinesiologist about my gut issues and had all of those injuries from running? I look back now and see how that moment was really the start of pursuing a functional way of life. Since then, I have committed a significant amount of time and energy to understanding more about the movement I do and the food I put in my body and how those choices impact the way I feel overall. I've also learned that my past does not have to dictate my present, nor does it have to determine my future. *We get to live in the present and be forward about our future.* And as a result of that shift in mindset, I've made some very big changes in my own life, including founding Alkalign as a company and, more importantly, adopting functional training as a way of life. More on that in a moment. First, let's talk about what it means to *live present, be forward.*

LIVE PRESENT

We've already established how the impact of food and fitness affects our physical health and sense of self. This impact is the fruit of seeds sown long ago by our culture, our upbringing, the media, our parents and caregivers, our peers, and so on. Every single one of those areas of influence have played a crucial role in what we believe to be true, about ourselves and the world around us. And my challenge to you has been to acknowledge and accept where you are right now with your food, your fitness, your deeply rooted beliefs, and your mindset. But there's a little more we need to talk about when it comes to mindset because, believe it or not, *you get to decide what you want for yourself going forward.*

A critical part of the mindset of living present and being forward is resetting the brain and re-informing the body about what it means to feel better from the inside out, rather than the outside in. One of my favorite authors, Brené Brown, has written, "When we deny the story, it defines us. When we own the story, we can write a brave new ending."[8] And the refreshing thing about the human brain is that it's a complex organ and acts like a muscle. The human brain is dynamic—it can contract and expand depending on input. Translation: *our brains can change.* The way we thought in the past doesn't have to be the way we think now. Because of our dynamic brain, it's never too late to shift our mindset and our lives.

MANAGING OUR MINDSET

When my firstborn, Ava, entered kindergarten, she was lucky to have an amazing teacher in a progressive public school where they focused on goals and educated the kids on having a growth mindset. Each week, Ava brought home a new growth-mindset mantra for the whole family to practice. Memorizing the mantras became a fun rhythm for our little family of four. We talked about them at dinner and in the car ride to and from school. Ava's favorite mantra was "Practice makes progress." Mine was "Whether you believe you can or you can't, you're right." Applying these growth-mindset mantras from her kindergarten class to my own life heightened my awareness of my own mindset and the mindsets of those around me. (Robert Fulghum was right on with his book *All I Really Need to Know I Learned in Kindergarten.*)[9] I started noticing how much mindset influenced outcomes for myself, my friends and family, and, especially, my employees and clients.

What I learned is that there are two types of mindsets: a *fixed* mindset and a *growth* mindset—essentially, the "I can't" versus the "I can." Another way to explain it is that the fixed mindset says, "this is the way it is and always will be because it always has been," and the growth mindset says, "that was then, this is now; tomorrow can be anything I want it to be." Do you see the difference?

In *Mindset: The New Psychology of Success*, psychologist Carol S. Dweck writes: "A fixed mindset comes from the belief that your qualities are carved in stone—who you are is who you are, period. Characteristics such as intelligence, personality, and creativity are fixed traits, rather than something that can be developed. A growth mindset comes from the belief that your basic qualities are things you can cultivate through effort. Yes, people differ greatly—in aptitude, talents, interests, or temperaments—but everyone can change and grow through application and experience."[10]

Another way to see the difference between the two mindsets is to think about them as roads. A fixed mindset is like a straight paved road. The behaviors are more rigid. It's a right-and-wrong, black-and-white way of thinking and living. A growth mindset is more of a meandering multi-surfaced path with many twists, turns, and potential destinations. It's a way of living where there are many possibilities to explore.

According to Dweck, we are all typically a combination of both mindsets. And much of who you are and how you show up in life on a day-to-day basis come from this combination. She also believes our mentalities can be seen as early as 4 years old. Four years old?!? Most of us probably have very few memories from age 4, yet so much of who we are was ingrained by that age. And this brings me back to my earlier point about belief systems. Not only were the seeds sown, but the way they were watered, fertilized, and nurtured has also greatly impacted the people we are today. If you identify as having a fixed mindset, you may feel a little hopeless right now, like you're locked into a specific destiny. But let this be your wakeup call, your opportunity to adopt a growth mindset and adapt things around you accordingly.

You might also be asking, *what does mindset have to do with health and wellness?* Everything. Before health is physical, it's behavioral. Labels such as *fat, skinny, smart, stupid, pretty, popular, teacher's pet* and *class clown* stick and can greatly impact our early sense of self. Our mindset influences our behaviors. The gravity of this reality weighs heavily as I'm raising two daughters who I'm desperately trying not to screw up. I'll be the first to admit there is a delicate balance between nurture and nature. We all have some genetic predispositions or tendencies deeply ingrained in our personalities, but even more ingrained are some of our experiences. How we harness those experiences and guide those tendencies makes a big difference in how we move forward.

The good news is that if behavior is learned, it can be relearned. As with our ability to develop physical strength or build endurance, we can change the course of our mindset over time. When we try something new, we get new feedback. This new feedback loop gives us new information, which eventually leads to a new mindset. That's why one of my new favorite mantras is "practice, not performance." Life is a *practice* where we work on progress, not a *performance* where we focus on perfection. This is also why *failure* is so important.

FEAR OF FAILURE

As a perfectionist, failure wasn't something I was comfortable with. In fact, I feared it. To me, failure was synonymous with weakness, pain, and unworthiness. Failure led to fear, and fear led to more failure. The only way to stop the incessant loop from going round and round was to completely reboot the system.

Rather than allow perfectionism to take over, I learned to exercise a growth mindset to face my fears head-on. Open water swimming, public speaking, and an entrepreneurial implosion of epic proportions were on the short list. The antidotes were swimming the shark-infested waters from Alcatraz to the San Francisco shore, taking up a secondary career as a fitness instructor where I had to wear a microphone and be in front of people, and opening a business that 99% of friends and family advised against. As scary as those experiences were, the outcomes weren't nearly as bad as the stories I had made up in my head. These experiences, combined with a series of small ones, retrained my brain to let go of perfection and fear of failure and embrace a growth mindset. Failure also gave me the gift of resilience. Things that used to devastate me now fall into the "this too shall pass" category. Besides, as Coach Mary always asks me, "what's the worst that can happen?"

Failure doesn't always have to hurt to work. The fear of failure is actually worse than failure itself, and the reward for persevering far outweighs the risk. In fact, failure isn't the problem; it's the speed at which we fail that takes us out of the game. We spend so much time agonizing over the perceived obstacles that we miss out on the opportunity to take advantage of the present. If we can learn to fail faster, then we retrain our brains to let failure work in our favor. When we fail fast, we have a greater capacity to pay attention to what's going on in us and around us, a greater capacity to *live present.*

PRACTICING MINDFULNESS

Pay attention is our No. 1 core value at Alkalign. Life moves quickly, so we encourage our clients with these words: *pay attention to you, pay attention to your surroundings, pay attention to those who you interact with on a daily basis, pay attention to how your actions and interactions impact the way you feel.* Paying attention is a simple and more direct way of communicating an ancient practice (also today's biggest buzzword): mindfulness.

Mindfulness is proven to have both physical and psychological benefits. Practicing mindfulness improves immunity,[11] reduces stress, regulates emotions, improves sleep, improves attention span and focus, reduces depression and anxiety,[12] and can assist in weight loss.[13] Almost sounds too good to be true, doesn't it? It's not. Mindfulness makes a difference. So why don't we practice it consistently all the time?

The reality is that mindfulness is easier said than done. It's challenging physically because we are used to moving a mile a minute, so slowing down and noticing is not in our modern-day DNA. And, psychologically, tuning in is tough because sometimes when we pay attention, we see things we don't like. We notice things we'd rather not. For me, this second part was especially tough given my good ole Irish Catholic way of life: *when you see something you don't like, you brush it under the rug and move on. If you pretend not to notice, no one else will, either.* Growing up with this mindset meant I was always moving. I kept busy with school, sports, and ballet. And I got annoyed at "slow" things, such as the pre-workout group stretch when I ran cross country and track. My life moved at mach speed without the opportunity, or the desire, to slow down. I never stopped to balance all of that intensity with something slow and mindful. This pattern continued into my mid-20s. I was either working crazy hours or training for something extreme. Occasionally, I'd attempt to slow down and take a Bikram yoga class. In reality, the 105-degree heat and 40% humidity of the studio was just another example of an extreme.

And although I truly could have benefited from the last few moments of savasana, the stillness was more than I could bear, so I'd sneak out early. Slowing down felt like the worst form of torture.

Mindfulness wasn't in my genes, or at least I didn't think so, until I experienced burnout from physical, emotional, and professional exhaustion. I couldn't keep pushing my body to the limits anymore. I needed to slow down and to reprioritize, not just once, but time and time again. First, I left banking. Then I left corporate America altogether. Then I stopped running. Then I moved beyond the barre to functional fitness. Slowly, I moved away from the parts of my past self that no longer served me and moved mindfully toward a new way of living. Like a snake shedding its skin, I sloughed off the layers I outgrew and made room in my life for more meaning.

But more important than these big moments of reprioritization are the little ones I make everyday. I now make time to read, meditate, gently move my body, and sleep. I nourish my body with nutrient-dense foods. I choose to look inward and pay attention to little things in life, such as the sounds of my kids' heartbeats and laughter when we snuggle each night. I notice how I move when I work out at Alkalign. I notice how my feet feel when I walk without shoes. I notice my posture when I'm driving in the car. I notice my breath throughout the day. I notice almost *everything* now, which is in stark contrast to my early days when I'd boast about how much I could "check out" and not think about anything while running endless miles. Now, as a result of paying attention, I'm actually more productive on any given day because I'm more mindful and more present.

Being mindful doesn't mean you have to be a Buddhist monk or adopt a serious meditation practice. You can find little ways to be mindful everyday. Mindfulness allows you to stay grounded and connect better to yourself. It's what allows you to *be forward* in the world around you.

BE FORWARD

When I talk about our mission to *live present, be forward,* what I mean is that today's actions impact tomorrow's outcomes.

For example, I inherited the idea that looking tan in my summer swimsuit was of utmost importance. Deep down, we all knew that too much sun exposure wasn't good, but it didn't stop me from actively prioritizing my tanning time during the prime hours of 10 a.m. and 2 p.m. whenever possible. My college roommates probably remember me dragging my Red Stripe-saturated body out of bed on spring break in Jamaica to get to the beach by 10 a.m. and staying until I was equally burned and blistered on both sides. I wasn't thinking about sunspots, sagging skin, premature aging, or potential melanoma. I wasn't thinking long term. I was thinking about the then and there. I prioritized the proverbial "here and now" because I'm human. And I enjoyed the instant gratification of tanned skin just as much as the next person, until I realized you can't separate the present from the future. You can't separate overexposure to the sun from skin damage in your 40s.

But bad habits are hard to change—unless we're willing to *live present* and *be forward.* Changing a habit isn't instant. It is more of a dimmer switch than a light switch that you can easily flip on and off. Modifying past habits, beliefs, and mindsets happens gradually over time. And the best way to not give up and go back to those bad habits is to set a few goals.

GO FOR THE GOAL

My kids are dumbfounded when I tell them I ate fast food and sugar cereal growing up. They can't believe that I would have ever avoided nuts, avocados, and butter because I believed fat of any kind was bad. They are even more wide eyed when I tell them that seat belts weren't the law when I was a kid and that car seats weren't a thing when their dad was a baby. My grandparents didn't understand the risks of smoking. My parents didn't initially understand the benefits of seat belts or sunscreen. I didn't understand the benefits of healthy fat for my brain. I didn't appreciate the damage that processed food would do to my microbiome or that running endless miles would do to my joints. It's not that any of us intend to put ourselves or our families in harm's way. In some cases, it is a lack of information and in others, lack of acceptance. As I've said before, *when you know better, you can do better.*

Studying my past was the wakeup call I needed for my own health. I honestly didn't notice how my previous actions impacted how I felt because I was moving too fast to pay attention or gain perspective. It wasn't until I was forced to take a step back to evaluate and identify past personal patterns that I was able to see the big picture, establish new habits, and go for the goal.

While understanding our health histories in order to be informed in the present is becoming more of a common practice, setting goals for our future is not. Think about it. When was the last time you did a vision board for your health? Perhaps you've crafted a vision board out of magazine cuttings for an event or a room in your house. These activities take place on Pinterest all day long. Yet I don't know anyone who has taken the time to write down goals for themselves for a greater vision of their health. Do you? I'm talking about goals such as "I want to improve my posture so I can avoid the neck and back pain associated with slumping over" or "I want to improve my foot alignment to avoid the ankle, knee, and hip pain that comes from walking, running, squatting, and lunging in improper alignment." Or "I want the strength and mobility to sit on, or get up from, the toilet without help when I'm 80." These goals may not be sexy or glamorous, but boy, being hunched over with back and neck pain or having someone else wipe your ass isn't exactly glamorous, either. But visioning for the future of our health requires something important we've already talked about. Yep, you guessed it: *it requires a change in mindset.* When you can change your past mindset and pay attention in the present, then you can set goals for a great vision of health in the future. This is how we *live present, be forward.*

My Challenge to You: Take a few moments to pause and look back at your past one last time. You may want to revisit past entries in your journal as you acknowledge the beliefs you have about food, fitness, sleep, stress management, and the concept of a healthy self in general. *Is there anything else you would add to those mindsets? Is there anything else you would add to the people, places, and patterns that have influenced your life up* *until this point?* There's no judgement in this challenge. A look at the past is what allows you to pay attention in the present. Consider your vision of health for the future. Are there goals you can establish now to help you reach your desired healthy future? Is there something you need to change in the present—something you could *stop* doing or *start* doing—in order to reach your desired future?

Find time this week to make a health vision board, in person or online, with images and quotes related to the life you want to be able to live 10 or 20 years from now. A functional approach to the future of our health can be attractive *and* practical. As my friend and mindfulness coach Lisa Abramson says, "When you own your story, you have an opportunity to write the ending." So let's start owning our stories and writing new endings today with the practice of health visioning.

GET A PhD IN YOU

"Knowing yourself is the beginning of all wisdom."

Aristotle

When I was growing up, I didn't think about the future in terms of my health, my joints, or my overall longevity. But it wasn't because I didn't care. Not caring isn't in my DNA. More likely, it was because I didn't know that it mattered. I didn't realize that the processed food I consumed was compromising the balance of good and bad bacteria in my gut microbiome. I didn't realize that the miles I ran were accelerating wear and tear on my joints. I had no idea 13 years of wedging my hips into unnatural positions in ballet would result in pelvic impairment. My crystal ball was more like a black Magic 8-Ball. My immature brain knew the immediate outcome it was looking for and I kept shaking the psychic sphere until I got the answer I wanted versus the one I needed. We all do this in our own ways. We have an amazing ability to talk ourselves into or out of anything we want. While I haven't been able to eradicate all of the deterioration in my body or fully recover from some unhealthy habits, I have come a long way, one small, healthy step at a time.

Bringing two girls into the world was another wakeup call. Suddenly, I realized that my lifestyle and my beliefs weren't just mine. They were something I would pass along to my girls, and I definitely didn't want to project my baggage and my poor food and exercise habits onto them. They didn't deserve that. But in order to truly share a healthier perspective with them, it had to start with me. I was the root of the messaging they would receive. I was the one they were watching, observing, and listening to at the most influential time in their lives. I had to reset my foundation so they could flourish. I had to envision a new future—one with confident kids who would grow up to love themselves and respect their bodies.

I went back to school for a degree in holistic nutrition and hired Coach Mary to help me blow up my own beliefs. I founded Alkalign in 2015 as a place that would be welcoming and supportive, no matter one's shape, size, or self-esteem. In doing so, I rewrote the health and wellness rules and worked around the clock to dispel the myths that constantly infiltrate our brains and flood our inboxes. I would live in a way that felt true and authentic to me, and if I could inspire someone along the way, that was a bonus. As much as I live for my girls, I realized I had to live for myself first. No one else could right the wrongs or mistakes from my past or love the unlovable parts of me. That had to come from within. I had to get a PhD in "me" in order to fully take charge and *be forward* about my life.

A PhD IN ME

As I always say and truly believe, no one should know you better than you. You are the person you spend the most time with. You are the person you have the most conversations with. You live with you and in you. All day. Every day. But like most things, the more we are "used" to something, like ourselves, the more we tend to tune it out or take it for granted. So *take a moment to get to know you.* How are you right now, really? No rote answers. You might need to put down the phone and power down the computer right now to focus on the one person you need in your life more than anyone. You. All of those other things in life that distract us from ourselves would cease to exist if it weren't for you. Your job, your children, your friends, your family, your faith, your pet, etc. What would they be without you? The world needs you, and the better you can show up, the better all those people who depend on you are going to be. In order to be there for others, you have to first be there for you. Think about your story—your thoughts, memories, and defining moments. Now think about what's important to you. Your family, health, financial security, career, relationships? How do they rank in theory versus in practice? Where would one be without the other? When you start uncovering these nuggets of inner wisdom, a clearer picture of *you* comes into focus.

How much you know about yourself depends on how much time you spend investing in the opportunity to study yourself. I'd like to think that we're all just a bunch of citizen scientists living our everyday lives. According to the UK-based Science Council, "a scientist is someone who systematically gathers and uses research and evidence to make hypotheses and test them, to gain and share understanding and knowledge."[14] Truth is, we don't have to wait for grad school or some professor to hand us a degree. We all have the potential to gather facts, organize knowledge, and to conduct experiments to improve our lives.

The combination of my academic background and my personal history coupled with years of experience working with human beings and bodies have given me a unique perspective. They've given me a PhD in me and the knowledge and perspective to guide you. Every single day at Alkalign, I watch, listen, and learn. I help my clients identify their mindset patterns just as much as their movement patterns. I recognize the progress they are making in their alignment and live for the shared joy of an "aha" moment. I can also see an injury or condition waiting to happen. But this didn't happen overnight. I first had to watch, listen, and learn about myself before I could do this for others.

You know when the personal PhD clicked for me? When I addressed my inner critic and understood the connection between the ego and the soul. Stay with me.

THE INNER CRITIC, THE EGO, AND THE SOUL

Have you ever struggled to feel good enough, smart enough, attractive enough, wealthy enough, fill-in-the-blank enough? Well, you can thank your inner critic for fueling that fire of fear. I remember when my inner critic, whom I affectionately call "Expectations Erin," first made herself known. I was 8 years old and focused on doing splits for my ballet teacher. Remember? She was the one who cared more about my perfect splits than my budding 8-year-old self-esteem or my future 80-year-old joints. At the same time, I cared more about pleasing people than I did about listening to my own body. All I could hear was Expectations Erin in my ear. Fast forward to the year I turned 40. There I was sitting in a personal development workshop learning about the inner critic and thinking back to the ballet story when it dawned on me that Ava was also 8 years old at the time. Did she already have an inner critic, too? I immediately went home and asked her if she had a little voice inside her head that ever told her she wasn't enough. Without even pausing, she described in great detail Angel Ava, Devil Ava, and Party Pooper Ava. Then she proceeded to draw this:

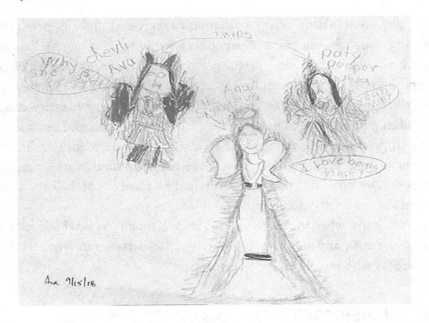

Wow. My dear sweet Ava had such wisdom at age 8. I did some research and found several studies supporting the findings that self-esteem peaks between ages 8–10 and falls off dramatically at age 12. Although puberty, the introduction of social media, and evolving social circumstances are likely the cause, the reality is depressing. The pressure was on. I only had a few more years to build up my daughter so she could tame her inner critic and be prepared to weather the storm of her tween and teen years. And yet at the same time, I knew I had to pay attention to my own inner critic so as not to beat myself up about everything that didn't go well in the parenting department. Ava and I agreed to work on it together. And thus, an awareness of our inner critic was introduced that has served as the foundation for our family-dinner-table discussions and conversations with my clients about their own inner dialogue, decision making, self-acceptance, self-love, and more.

Here's what I want you to know: *we all have an inner critic.* And as much as I am a huge fan of self-care and self-reflection, I also believe in not overanalyzing or allowing your worst enemy to live between your ears. The hardest part about embarking on something new is the battle we wage within ourselves. And the inner critic isn't the only thing at play.

The ego and the soul are in there, too. Everyone has all three of them in different proportions and at different times in life. We'll get to the ego and the soul soon, but let's stick with the inner critic right now. I see the struggle we all have with our inner critic every day in my business. The inner critic is constantly yapping in our ear about how we can't do something or why we won't do it well enough. It's the voice that tells us we are bad, wrong, inadequate, or even worthless. It instills fear, which robs us of our opportunity to explore, to evolve, and to enjoy the present and all it has to offer. It's also the No. 1 reason people don't walk in my studio doors; they are intimidated by what their inner critic has to say.

So much of what we fear is thanks to our inner critic. And so much of what we are drawn to is ego driven. The line between our inner critic and our ego is the constant back and forth between what we want and what we think we do or do not deserve. We want to be fit, but we're not sure we really deserve it. So we push our body until it hurts with high-intensity exercises such as running, CrossFit, extreme training, and competitive court sports even when our knees are about to give out. It's the "more is more" mindset. Conversely, there are people who want to be fit but are not really sure if they are capable, so they lean out of fitness altogether. Both responses come from the same desire—*to be fit*—and the same inner-critic message—*we don't deserve it*. While the behaviors look different, the motivations are the same.

So what is the ego? Latin for *I*, it's what drives us to care about the things we think we should have and the things we think we deserve: a beautiful outward appearance (often at the expense of inner health), a big bank account, a brand new house, a nice car, a successful career, perfectly executed birth plans, the best school for our kids to attend. These things aren't bad in and of themselves. What can get messy is our mindset toward these things. And that mindset is driven by our ego. We all have an ego, each of us to differing degrees. According to purpose coach Tim Kelley, author of *True Purpose*, "our thoughts, our feelings, our ability to make choices, are all contained within the ego. It contains everything we know about ourselves and the world around us." Kelley explains that the ego is the "conscious," and it functions according to a set of values intended to make us feel good, protect us, and help us survive and thrive. In general, the ego values health, money, and happiness and avoids fear, pain, and struggle. It divides our experiences into good and bad, or likes and dislikes. Our egos are why we crave a particular life status, like owning a home and a fast car, living in a specific place, and being in a committed, loving relationship. Because of our egos, we long for acceptance, approval, admiration, and respect from others. We are concerned about how others perceive us and what they think about us.[15] Sound familiar?

In contrast, Kelley describes the soul as the "part of us that guides us along our life's path . . . that part of you that already knows your purpose in life." The soul is the "'unconscious,' the things we do not know.'" He goes on to describe the values of the soul as concerned with *being*, not *doing* (in contrast to the ego). Kelley says the soul has a long-term view of life and no preference for what experience the ego is having. The soul doesn't divide experiences into good and bad. In fact, it doesn't divide anything up into categories like the ego does. Rather, the soul sees our lives as a work of art or journey. So what's its purpose? The main function of the soul is to guide the development of the ego. Our soul influences our decisions and helps us choose things that will develop us in ways that serve our purpose rather than succumb to the latest pleasure. According to the soul, all experiences are learning opportunities along the path of life, no matter how the ego experiences them. Kelley further differentiates the two. The soul "is concerned with how we learn and grow from our experiences, not with whether or not we like them."[16]

My life experience has taught me what studies show—that life is good when the ego is kept in balance or in check by the soul.[17] But things are rarely ever in perfect balance. That's why it's important to tune in and notice what is going on and keep the ego and the soul away from the extremes on either end of the spectrum. To really get a PhD in you, your soul must be present and active alongside your ego. And here's why this is really, really important: *the modern-day health and wellness industry preys on your ego.* The promises of faster, thinner, stronger, sweatier, happier, or wealthier with the latest products are low-hanging fruit for industry marketers. When your ego is out of check, it will be easy to take your eyes off of what you know to be true and best for you and believe what some random tagline tells you.

The fitness industry is ego dominant because that's the easy sell. People want to buy the promise, not the process. Promise is ego. Process is soul. By now you're probably curious how I would categorize exercise programs between the ego and the soul. Since finding the right kind of movement and learning to balance the ego and the soul is helpful for the PhD in you, here are a few exercise programs I would consider ego dominant: CrossFit, performance-based boot camps, and activities focused on extrinsic goals and external metrics such as amount of weight used, wattage recorded, number of reps completed, and heart rate and caloric burn achieved. With the rising popularity of smart watches and biohacking gadgets, almost any workout can become ego dominant if the participant is working in that frame of mind. Ironically, one of the most obviously ego-dominant workouts put *soul* in its name. It markets the soul all the while preying on the ego.

Ego is what buys the promise of the hot bod that will result from these activities. Ego is what convinces you it's acceptable to subscribe to a workout that recommends two hours of equal parts hot and humid exercise a day to look a certain way. In contrast, yoga is generally considered a more soul-dominant practice because of its historically spiritual roots. However, yoga has been ego-fied in more recent years with the introduction of hot yoga, power yoga, and the promotion of everything in the extreme, including backbends, handstands, hypermobility, and megalomaniacal "gurus." I've seen a lot of clients end up really jacked up because their ego took over in yoga.

The bottom line is that we all have an inner critic, an ego, and a soul. The ego isn't necessarily "bad," but it can push us to the extreme if left on its own. My advice: name the inner critic (you gotta name it to tame it), and, like the 80s waffle commercial implored us, "leggo the ego"—not entirely, but at least dial it back to create more space for your soul. Doing so will create clarity around your purpose in life. And when you find your purpose, you will feel fulfilled, passionate, and like you're making a difference—because you really *are* making a difference. This is what I call *alignment in your life.* Letting go of the ego is also what it takes to get a PhD in you. Are you ready to do the research?

Important sidenote: While I'm not into figuring out the newest tracking features of the latest smartwatches, I do own a Fitbit. (I'm telling you here because I don't want you to think I'm a hypocrite.) My Fitbit arrived thanks to a family fitness challenge I did with my kids at the height of the COVID-19 pandemic in 2020. It was the motivation we all needed to get moving after sheltering in place at home for months on end. But I was aware that I had to be really careful and keep my "tracking" ego in check. So my soul owns that Fitbit, not my ego. However, almost immediately, my youngest daughter, Elle, was motivated to move by the device and equally unmotivated to move when it was out of battery life. Raising kids whose eyes and ears are ever curious, I'm very careful not to send the wrong messages. At the same time, I want to plant seeds that will help them flourish into confident, thriving, healthy humans who spend their precious lives *enjoying life* instead of fretting over what they eat, how they look, or how many workouts they did. Movement doesn't have to be measured in order for it to be meaningful, nor does anything else.

My Challenge to You: Do your own research about you. Take an assessment of what's working and not working when it comes to food, fitness, overall health, and lifestyle choices. If you have no idea, then start tracking your workouts, your meals, your hormone changes, and how you feel on a consistent basis—with your soul, not your ego. There's always an app for stuff like that, or you can pull out your journal and jot it down there. *What changes do you need to make, and what steps will you take to make those changes?* Note: When I got to this point in my PhD in me, I started searching for health practitioners who understood an integrated, functional approach to a holistic life, like how nutrition affects my exercise, how exercise affects my everyday movements, and how my mental and emotional well-being comes into play, too. So do your research on you, and then do your research on who can be a part of the team taking care of you.

PRINCIPLE SEVEN:
DO THE BEST WITH WHAT YOU'VE GOT

"We don't see things as they are.
We see them as we are."

Anais Nin

O ne of the things I catch myself saying out loud to my friends, clients, and even my own kids is: *we can't control what happens in the universe, but we can control how we respond to it*. This reality comes from a combination of mindset and mechanics, meaning what we *think* and how we *act* are a result of our beliefs. It's not to say that a proactive, preventative person can't get caught off guard by difficult circumstances. Because as much as you try, you certainly can't prevent all fires in life. In 2021 alone, I've said goodbye to three friends whose long and arduous battles with various forms of cancer couldn't be stopped with all of the proactive, preventative measures each one had in place. But barring tragedies such as cancer, the magnitude, frequency, and impact of our everyday life incidents can be minimized when we're willing to think critically and make the investment in ourselves to preserve and protect our bodies and our well-being.

Throughout my life, I have had to show up for myself time and time again, just like you've had to do for yourself. My journey of self-exploration and self-care has made me who I am and has inspired me to help others be their best selves, too. Along the way, my mindset has shifted as I've learned about and accepted my mechanics. I know that my body isn't "perfect." I will always have cellulite, sunspots, gray hair, and jiggly bits. But I also have hands and feet that keep me steady and grounded, legs that allow me to walk and dance (and boy, do I love to dance!), arms that allow me to cook and hug, a brain that allows me to think for myself, and a strong mind that allows me to make decisions for myself. My body is the only body I'm ever going to have, and I'm committed to taking care of it, from the inside out. This means I'm going to do the best with what I've got, and I want the same for you, too.

So here are 7 tips for doing the best with what you've got:

THINK CRITICALLY (WITHOUT BEING CRITICAL)

If running made you fat, would you still do it? If kale were terrible for you, would you still eat it? Chances are you might still do it if you had heard a thousand times before that both options were good for you. That's the power of marketing. It's also the absence of critical thinking.

Did you know that we think about 6,000 thoughts a day and these thoughts may be repeated day after day?[18] These repetitive thoughts create repetitive patterns, which create the experiences of our lives. So if your thoughts are continuously negative, self-limiting, and/or self-diminishing, those are the patterns you repeat in your everyday life experiences. If your thoughts are life-giving, creative, and radiant, then those are the patterns that pop up for you in your experiences. If you want to change your mindset from negative thinking to positive thinking, you have to *think critically*. According to the Foundation for Critical Thinking, to think critically means to use "that mode of thinking ... in which the thinker improves the quality of his or her thinking by skillfully taking charge of the structures inherent in thinking and imposing intellectual standards upon them." This is done by "conceptualizing, applying, analyzing, synthesizing, and/or evaluating information." It is "self-directed, self-disciplined, self-monitored, and self-corrective thinking."[19] Critical thinking means considering standards of excellence, mindfulness, communication, and problem-solving abilities and implies a commitment to be less egocentric, as is our human tendency. If you think critically about whether extreme running, or extreme exercise of any kind, is good for you, chances are you might change the way you exercise. And if you think critically about the food you need to nourish your body, you might change the way you eat.

The truth is it's easy to get caught in a rut of routine, comfort, and complacency. Back when I was running everyday, I actually found peace in the mindless movement. Running was like a metronome that kept me on course. Although the miles were causing discomfort in my physical body, the trance-like routine and familiarity were soothing for my psyche. I told myself that it was what I needed for my mental and physical health. I convinced myself that extreme cardio was the only option and that because I was so intense in other areas of my life, personally and professionally, I had to match that with something as intense to "let off steam." Really, I needed to counterbalance my intensity in some way, but it would take me a while to think this way. Even when I began making big strides in other aspects of my life, such as my career and my gut health, I held tight to my runner's identity. I stayed the course because it seemed less scary than steering the ship in a different direction. Returning to my repetitive thoughts and equally repetitive (and competitive) actions was easier than accepting the alternative—having to wake up and think for myself. That's why for years Coach Mary has challenged me at every decision intersection with a version of the famed question coined by *Loving What Is* author Byron Katie: "Is it true?" When I stop and ask, *is it true?* about my assumptions and repetitive thought patterns, I'm forced to think critically and change my mindset around any unhealthy assumptions, which, left unchecked, turn into accusations.

And here's what I finally learned after thinking critically about food and fitness. It changed me and has the power to change you, too: *What worked for someone you know may not work for you. And what worked for you two months, two years, or two decades ago most likely won't work for you now.*

As humans, we are ever-evolving. Part of evolving is learning, and learning requires critical thinking. Take food fads, for instance. Food fads are easy to believe if we're not doing our research. Believe me, I've tried all the diets from cabbage soup to Keto. I've counted calories, carbs, and kilos, all the while convincing myself that I could somehow magically outsmart the body I was given. But those fads didn't work as promised. And everytime I got to the end of a fad, I felt worse than when I started. Now when up against a fad, I do my research and compare it to the functional nutrition method I currently use to take care of my body.

Functional nutrition is all about nourishing your body with the nutrients it needs to thrive. I eat as many unprocessed or minimally processed foods as possible and try to reduce the consumption of foods made in a packaged goods factory. I try to eat like author Michael Pollan advises in *In Defense of Food*: "Eat food. Not too much. Mostly plants."[20] Functional nutrition is nothing fancy. In fact, it's the simplicity that is effective and timeless. Once I went back to the basics and embraced not being beholden to the newest diet craze, I was actually able to stop obsessing about or fearing the effects of food and start enjoying it. My shift from running to exercising in a different way was similar to my breakup with fad dieting. I took something natural for humans, the movement of running, to the very extreme. And modern inventions, like running shoes and supportive orthotics, allowed me to keep doing it. But my body was telling me that the running I was doing was too much, too fast, as evidenced by the injuries I experienced on a regular basis. In addition to the hip replacement warning that rocked me to the core, thinking critically and knowing that I couldn't out-evolve evolution brought me back to everyday movements that were good for my body. Thinking critically brought me back to functional fitness.

Quick sidenote: not all fads are bad. Some are innocuous. Take bell bottoms, permed hair, and blue eyeshadow. Aside from an embarrassing photo resurfacing decades later, those fashion fads aren't going to hurt you. As I write this book, I believe that the blue-light glasses I'm wearing, perhaps another fad, are somehow helping to save my eyes from excessive screen time or at least are not causing additional harm. When I think critically about it, I know there is no way this plastic lens could possibly offset the accelerated impact modern technology has had on my eyes compared to their intended, natural evolution. But, alas, wearing the glasses makes me feel better. It makes me feel like I'm at least doing something to help myself. The challenge with food and fitness fads is being able to see through the excitement of the "here and now" to evaluate risk versus reward. Is one Snackwell cookie or CrossFit class going to kill you? Probably not. But it's not doing you much good, either, especially when the mindset that comes with believing you have to eat and exercise according to the marketing machines overtakes your ability to think critically.

When I was growing up, my father used to say, "if you've taught your children to think for themselves, you've taught them everything." And I think it's safe to say my parents succeeded. I'm grateful for the experiences and challenges I had and the confidence and sense of self I developed as a result. Thinking critically is what gave me the courage to move away from harmful food and fitness fads and see the whole industry in a different light. It has allowed me to understand myself and others in a different way. It has inspired me to help more people explore, understand, and potentially disrupt their repetitive thought patterns so they can learn to think critically, too. Even though I am proud of where

I am, I sometimes wonder what I could have experienced or contributed to the world if I hadn't wasted so many of my thoughts and my time on how I could best conform to societal expectations. *What if some of my energy had been redirected elsewhere, and earlier?* I hope my regret is an encouragement to you, that it helps you pause and think about what you could do if you had less fear, worry, and stress.

If this doesn't make you want to look at life through a different lens, then consider the costs of staying where you are. That cost comes in the form of *denial*. What I know now, after years of research, education, and my own therapy journey, is that denial is a defense mechanism. I also think it was the root cause of all of my gut and injury issues, too. According to the Mayo Clinic: "Denial is a coping mechanism that gives you time to adjust to distressing situations—but staying in denial can interfere with treatment or your ability to tackle challenges. If you're in denial, you're trying to protect yourself by refusing to accept the truth about something that's happening in your life. In some cases, initial short-term denial can be a good thing, giving you time to adjust to a painful or stressful issue. It might also be a precursor to making some sort of change in your life. But denial has a dark side."[21] I've felt trapped on that dark side many times and, simultaneously, too paralyzed by fear to peek my head out and search for something else.

Denial exists for all of us in one form or another. Whether it's the workout you're convinced is good for you or the Diet Coke that definitely "doesn't cause cancer," we choose to believe what we want to believe and what our thought patterns want to repeat. And as free-willed humans, we can make whatever choices we want to make about our bodies and our lives. But the rub is that with great freedom comes great responsibility. You have been gifted *one* body and *one* life. You, and only you, have a great responsibility to take good care of your body with proper nutrition that nourishes your body and exercise movements that support and strengthen your body for the long haul. I'm not saying you should forever avoid the things you love. An occasional Diet Coke isn't going to kill you. Rather, I recommend moderation and balancing out the effects of your passions with the practical.

For example, if you enjoy a higher risk activity for your joints such as tennis, skiing, or running, consider cross-training to improve your alignment and strengthen your muscles. If you are running, boxing, or jump squatting to blow off steam, recognize that you are also stressing your body. In my experience, balancing the intensity of your favorite activity with something like a self-massage rolling class, meditation, or strength and conditioning goes a long way. Too much of a good thing usually isn't good, especially if it's out of balance. That's why CrossFit is initially appealing. It's built on a functional philosophy, but in practice CrossFit easily becomes too extreme. If your body is so jacked up that you need a jackhammer-like tool such as a Theragun to undo the damage, it's probably a sign that the activities or lifestyle that got you in that pickle is not sustainable. At the end of the day, denial is a choice, and if you choose it, consequences are inevitable. But when you choose to think critically about your choices, you no longer use denial as a coping mechanism.

Here's the last thing I'll say about thinking critically. Sometimes we have the opportunity to benefit from the lessons we learn from others. Those of us who have access to a family medical history have a crystal ball of sorts. We at least know some of our risk factors, and these can influence our everyday choices. For example, I'm at high risk for a variety of lovely things such as colon cancer, aortic aneurysms, and Dupuytren's contracture, a condition when your hands fold into themselves and become claw-like. As depressing as these things are, I'm grateful to have this knowledge because I'm a prevention person. I had my first colonoscopy at age 35. I took a test for aneurysms and will continue to be monitored via regular ultrasounds after the age of 60. And when it comes to the hands, I roll my hands with massage therapy balls regularly to keep them mobile. I also take global measures to reduce inflammation in my body as inflammation is the root cause of disease.[22] I have no idea if I will inherit any of these afflictions. What I do know is that at some point something will go awry. It always does. And while an eventual breakdown is inevitable, I can choose to prepare my body and mind to offset the impact as much as possible. I decided to make a choice while I had a choice.

Sound overwhelming? Probably. And that's OK. Start where you are, and do the best with what you've got. Remember, my prevention mindset didn't manifest overnight. It came from a reflection on how I was using denial as a defense mechanism, and it came from outside help with identifying what's important to me and what I'm willing to invest in the future of my health. And even though I'm all about practicing prevention, there are a number of things I'm not willing to give up entirely in my life, such as dark chocolate. If you said I could give up dark chocolate and live to 120, I'd opt for a shorter lifespan (remember, *practices, not performances*). Life is about choices. I choose chocolate. But I do so thinking critically.

UNDERSTAND YOUR BIO-INDIVIDUALITY

In my fitness studios, we talk about learning styles, meaning that people learn in different ways: visual, auditory, and somatic (or kinesthetic). I am a somatic learner, which means, for me, physically feeling something is believing it. For visual learners, they have to see it to believe it, and auditory learners have to hear it to believe it. As a somatic or kinesthetic learner, I had to feel the difference functional movement made in my body before I was willing to embrace it. I had to try a few rolling exercises and feel how my body responded before I was sold on Jill Miller's *Roll Model* method. I had to try many different ways of eating before I found what worked for me and became convinced that I should stick with it versus constantly seeking the "next best thing." I had to feel my way to change, one adaptation and one day at a time. But it might be different from you, and that's OK. That's all part of our *bio-individuality*. Bio-Individuality is a term coined by Joshua Rosenthal, founder of the Institute for Integrative Nutrition, where I received my health coaching and hormone health certifications. Bio-individuality recognizes that each individual body differs in nutrition and fitness needs as a result of our external and internal factors like the foods we eat, our emotional thoughts, our lifestyle patterns, our physical environment, and the ways we move our bodies. As Rosenthal explains it, "Bio-individuality means that no one diet works for everyone. Each and every person has unique needs."[23]

In addition to bio-individuality, we also have to consider our *biomechanics.* Biomechanics is the science that studies the mechanics of human movement and includes the components of motion, force, momentum, levers, and balance. As you can imagine, these factors are critical in understanding how your unique body works. One of the best ways to improve your physical fitness is to acquire a deeper understanding of how the body moves and the capacity of joints, bones, and ligaments to perform certain actions. Individuals who incorporate proper biomechanics are able to pursue their potential to its highest level and help minimize the risk of injury. Professional athletes and weekend warriors alike can benefit from this knowledge and even more so from putting it into practice. But have no fear. You don't have to go back and get a degree in biophysics to improve your life. There are many resources you can leverage to learn more about your body and how it works. My personal favorites are *Move Your DNA* and *Whole Body Barefoot*, both by biomechanist Katy Bowman, and, fortunately, both are fun and not written like a boring science book.

Among bio-individuality, biomechanics, and individual learning styles, there is an incredible amount of variation that exists in the human body and human brain. This is one of the reasons it's important for us to listen to what our individual bodies are telling us.

LEARN YOUR BODY'S LANGUAGE

Human movement is universal, and because of this, it's something most of us don't fully understand or really ever think about. We don't have to take classes to learn how to roll over, crawl, walk, or run. We don't have to learn to breathe, eat, or eliminate. By default, it all happens naturally. But at some point, we are forced to engage and learn more about our body and our movements. Whether it is a simple sprain or a major joint replacement, we pause and pay attention to how our movement affects our bodies.

The hard part is we think we already know everything about our bodies because human movement is one of our native languages. But even native speakers of a language have to go to school to learn the mechanics of their language—grammar, spelling, etc.—because language is complex. The human body is equally complex, and learning about it is like taking a language arts class. Learning about *your body* is like analyzing your unique way of speaking English: it's your dialect plus your accent and word choice. No two people speak exactly the same way, just as no two bodies are exactly alike thanks to bio-individuality, which means each human has unique needs based on internal and external factors. Yet despite all this complexity, our bodies do not come with an owner's manual, nor do we go to school to learn how to operate them day to day. Even if we take anatomy to study body systems and parts or learn about movement in P.E. class or sports, we are rarely taught the mechanics of how things work and how the expression of movement or our food consumption impacts the functionality of our everyday lives. We take our movement and our health for granted until something goes wrong, at which point we rely on someone else to "fix it." In some cases, we may end up in a nutritionist's office, on a surgeon's operating table, or in physical therapy to re-learn what was lost, but preventative learning on how to avoid such issues, especially learning tailored to a person's bio-identity, is almost *nonexistent.*

The more I learn about the human body and the being within it, the more I realize there is no substitute for the human experience, both mine and yours. Yes, it's helpful to know the basics of human anatomy, biomechanics, and functional nutrition. It's why we teach so many of these principles at Alkalign in a way that is both nutritious and digestible for the whole you. Our job is to educate, empower, and inspire you, but that's only helpful if you pay attention to your own human experience— how your own unique body moves and feels and what you sense your unique body needs. I might have made different decisions in my teens and 20s had I known that it doesn't have to hurt to work—if I knew that my injuries were a sign that excessive running was accelerating the wear and tear on my unique body and that fat-free eating was perpetuating poor gut health for my unique and extremely sensitive digestive system. It's possible I was never cut out for running, or perhaps I was never taught the proper biomechanics of running. Or maybe I just overdid it and didn't have the core strength and alignment principles to offset the damage I was doing to my body.

And I could say something similar for my gut health. I wish I knew back then that it was OK to order *off-menu* when I was out to eat at a restaurant or having dinner with friends. The best way to explain what I mean by ordering off-menu is from the movie *When Harry Met Sally:*

> "But I'd like the pie heated, and I don't want the ice cream on top. I want it on the side, and I'd like strawberry instead of vanilla if you have it. If not, then no ice cream, just whipped cream, but only if it's real. If it's out of the can, then nothing."

I now know that what I put into my body makes a difference in how I feel, and I want to make informed decisions by picking the best food options for *me*—options that nourish my individual body. If you've ever been to a restaurant, coffee shop, or juice bar with me, you know I love to inquire about everything, from the nutritional content of ingredients to the preparation. I ask a plethora of questions, secretly wondering if the waitstaff thinks I'm the "worst" kind of customer. I'd like to think I'm low maintenance, but I'm sure there have been a few servers who have called me otherwise. But the truth is, I enjoy engaging and interacting with the human on the other side of my complex order versus feeling like it's a one-way transaction.

I also no longer believe there is *one way* to eat, or even exercise, for all of humankind at any given time. That's why we have different menu options. Some customizations are a preference; others are required for true optimization for the individual. For example, consider my order at In-N-Out Burger, my preferred drive-through-style restaurant when on a road trip. The restaurant has a whole "secret" menu that allows you to customize your burger until it's *just right*. I order my burger "animal style" and "protein style." While my request for "animal style" (caramelized onions, pickles, and extra special sauce) is a *preference*, my request for "protein style" (in a lettuce wrap instead of a bun) is a *necessity* because my gut does not feel good when gluten is involved. This takes me back to something Ann Wigmore, a pioneer of natural health, wrote, "The food you eat can be either the safest and most powerful form of medicine or the slowest form of poison."[24] Let that soak in for a minute.

Nut free, dairy free, gluten free. These may seem like ridiculous requests, but for people who have issues or allergies, they are very real. Variation exists in so many things including religious preference and skin tone, body mechanics and microbiome, so why not food? It took me a long time to figure out that variation is a real thing just like it took me a long time to embrace it in myself. Once I did, I was never able to go back to ordering off of the menu. Now I order *off-menu*, and I'm OK with embracing Goldilocks-style meals wherever we go.

Only *you* live in your body. Only *you* are responsible for taking care of it and ensuring it gets what it needs to thrive. A special *off-menu* order doesn't make you "high maintenance"; it makes you informed about what's best for *you*. And that is one of the greatest gifts you can give to yourself—making the best choices you can for your particular body. So embrace your advanced understanding of you and your body's language, and celebrate how much better you feel as a result.

The bottom line is that bio-individuality means we need to make unique decisions on what's best for our individual bodies—not based on the latest fads or what seems to be best for the masses. You deserve a better understanding of *you*.

PRESERVE, PROTECT, INVEST

Now that I'm a self-labeled preventionist, I do my best to find health practitioners who think the same way—with a prevention mindset. A few years ago, I was in search of a new general physician after being in a monogamous relationship with my OB–GYN during my child-birthing years. The search felt a little like an awkward round of doctor speed-dating. First, I went to an internist. During the intake appointment, I told her that I believe lifestyle greatly influences my overall well-being. Given my years of trial and error with my own body, particularly my gut health, I had firsthand experience in how everyday choices impacted everyday outcomes. She responded with, "My job is to fix things when they break." That's it. There was nothing else as a transition to the kind of preventative practice I was hoping to hear about that day. I wanted to hear her talk about how important it was to preserve and protect our bodies and invest in our health with preventative practices. But it was evident from our brief exchange that we had different approaches, and I promptly added myself to a different waitlist to see an integrative medicine specialist who was, indeed, a much better fit.

Pursuing preventative medicine rather than reacting to injuries and pain in the moment takes thoughtful, proactive consideration. It also requires an understanding that different things work for different people. The ways we preserve and protect our bodies as investments will be individual and unique for every person. There is no "one size fits all" when it comes to preventative medicine. And it's important to find health practitioners who share similar beliefs and are willing to partner with you to put those approaches into practice.

Beyond finding an integrative health specialist, a holistic and functional approach was the answer to the question I had been asking, *how can I strike a balance between maintaining my body now and preserving it for later?* I realized I was caught up in all the fitness fads because I believed I had to live for today. I was living for the numbers on my scale, which directly correlated to my sense of self. I disregarded the benefits of my strong body and athletic build and instead sought the "skinny" status in a society that praised that extreme and punished the other. Besides, *who cares about tomorrow?* Who cares if I starve myself to the point of interfering with my future fertility? Who cares if I initiate a snowball of hormonal health issues that will interfere with life for decades to come? Well, it turns out I did. I used to believe "if it ain't broken, why fix it?" Then I broke, and I desperately wanted to fix it, right away and for my future. I wanted a physical and mental breakthrough from my chains and was willing to abandon the fads I had religiously followed to get it.

In reality, the health and wellness industry does not run on accountability, willpower, premeditated plans, or self-directed sustainable solutions. The COVID-19 crisis is a good example of this. It was overlooked for a long time. Like everything else, we thought we could brush it under the rug and it would go away. When it didn't, we sought human nature's second line of defense, an instant fix. COVID-19 is an extreme example of what happens when planning and foresight are extremely overlooked. A little bit of foresight, funding, and mindful leadership could have gone a long way in proactively preparing the world for a pandemic of epic proportions. But, like anything else, you can't change what was. You can only impact what is. How you respond on a micro level to macro circumstances matters.

While your personal fitness and nutrition perspective pales in comparison to something as massively consequential as the coronavirus, the basic principles still apply. There is no substitute for awareness and prevention, nor is there a replacement for personal responsibility. When it comes to your health, you are the one responsible for preserving and protecting your body. You are the one responsible for your outcome, and your outcome is only as good as your investment. And that investment yield is more like a treasury bond than a rapidly rising tech stock. Generally speaking, the faster the rise, the harder the fall. Slow and steady wins the race when it comes to your health and wellness if you're in it for the long game. And the long game of slow fitness and slow, nutritious food is how you preserve and protect your body as an investment. It's not only important to know where you are today, but also to know where you want to be tomorrow.

KNOW YOUR ENDGAME

Speaking of goals, it was in a 2009 childbirth prep class that I finally learned the difference between a plan and a goal. Sarah McMoyler, a labor and delivery RN, cautioned the eager, type A, soon-to-be new parents in the room to avoid the "birth plan." She said, "you can have goals, but there is no such thing as a plan." What she meant was I needed a broad plan focused on overarching goals, rather than a prescriptive plan focused on detailed steps of the process. I didn't realize it at the time, but this was the most impactful advice for parenting, business, and life in general that I've ever received.

In the case of childbirth, the overarching goal and ultimate plan is *"healthy baby, healthy mom."* Yet so many of us go into pregnancy and childbirth with expectations. We try to dictate the story and control the experience before it even takes place. We want the home birth, the natural birth, the silent birth, the unicorn and rainbows birth. Who knows where these expectations come from—the media, parents, friends, the *Bible*, a celebrity? Ultimately, it doesn't matter where they come from because, like many other things, they are so deeply rooted that we can't change how they got there. But we can change what we do with them. Sarah did this for me. She planted a seed that inspired a shift in mindset about my birth "plan."

Two months after that birthing class, Ava decided it was time to arrive. It was a very uneventful Saturday. I woke up ten days before my due date, got dressed to work out, and sat on the toilet to pee. When things lingered like the "evacuation complete" scene from the first *Austin Powers* movie, I realized it wasn't due to being super hydrated, but, rather, my water had broken. I packed my stability ball and headed to the hospital to push out that baby. I knew I was 100% on board for the epidural. I had seen the brutal videos of the drug-free births, and I didn't want to punch Tony in the face if things got ugly.

Surprisingly, I didn't have a specific birth plan typed out in a spreadsheet like I did for every other life event. But not so surprisingly, deep down I had some big expectations. I thought that because I was in great shape, had wide hips, and good genes from my mom—who naturally birthed 4 children on her own—that I would have a very easy vaginal delivery. I fully expected (and desperately wanted) to be the poster child for an easy childbirth. But 16 hours of labor and 1 ½ hours of pushing later, Dr. O called it. I was headed into surgery for an emergency C-section. Apparently, I wasn't making any progress due to an odd-shaped pelvis despite my "high quality" functional pushing. Ava's heart rate was dropping, and they had to get her out. I could sense the stress in the room and knew it wasn't good. Despite being drugged and delirious, I vividly remember the way Dr. O delivered the news. She apologized profusely: "Erin, I'm so sorry, but we have to do a C-section. I know how hard you've worked for those abs!" I chuckled. Her humor lightened the mood. But I was fine with the decision. At that moment, I couldn't have cared less about my abs or my appearance. I just kept thinking, *healthy baby, healthy mom.* Plan A (a vaginal delivery) didn't work out. But because I stayed focused on the goal versus "the plan," I could easily shift gears and not stay stuck on the original birth expectations. Thirty minutes later, Ava was born, and Tony's nose was still intact. Mission (and goal) accomplished.

MAKE IT FUNCTIONAL

My personal and professional mission is to inspire wellness on a whole different level. That's why I care about helping you find freedom in your life, too. But I honestly don't think that many people who walk in the doors of my fitness studios can pinpoint why they are there. Initially, they come for the "check-the-box" workout experience we've all been conditioned to crave. But they stay because the experience is so much more. Alkalign becomes a lifestyle for them.

Exercise is an important component, and it's the vehicle that allows our bodies to deliver so much more on a daily basis. Functional fitness specifically is designed to train your body for day-to-day activities. Even then, "exercise" is just one component in the greater picture of functional living. Behind the fitness classes and nutrition coaching of Alkalign is a very intentional goal: to motivate clients to be the superhero of their own life story. It's the reason the Alkalign logo has a super-hero-style letter A. That was no accident. We take the shame, blame, and swimsuit references out of the equation and replace that messed-up messaging of fast fitness and fake food with a safe, sustainable, and science-based approach to human health. That's why we go back to the basics with functional movement. Because we recognize that, at the end of the day, the simple joy of being able to squat, walk, sit, and stand without pain is not something to take for granted. These are the very same movements you employ in some way each and every day. You might as well learn to do them well as you find freedom in functional movement.

For a quick recap, the seven "official" functional movements are

squatting, hinging, lunging, pushing, pulling, rotating, and **walking**. Each time you sit on the toilet you are *squatting*. Each time you open the refrigerator or car door you are *pulling*. Each time you mow the lawn, shop with a cart, or walk with a stroller, you are *pushing*. Each time you reach to the back seat to get something from your bag you are *rotating*. Each time you bend over to spit out your toothpaste or pick something up you are *hinging*. And with every step you take, you are practicing the asymmetrical principles of both *lunging* and *walking*.

These examples may not seem all that glamorous, but imagine life without being able to do any of these seven essential movements. If you've ever had an injury, even something as minor as a stubbed toe, you have learned to appreciate when everything works properly and how everything in the body is connected. Even a stubbed pinky toe leads to a change in gait, or the way you walk. A change in gait leads to an imbalance in the hips, which leads to increased load in the lower back, and so on. I think you get the picture. The purpose of functional training is to recognize that all parts are important and if we want the parts to last, we have to practice taking care of them. Like doing anything in life, the more you hone a craft, the better you get. The more you purposefully practice functional movement, the more smoothly you walk or run through life, free of the injuries and issues that otherwise inevitably impact your ability to move, live, and be. And the better you move, the more fun you can have in life. Functional sounds boring, but if you do it right, it's anything but.

Functional living is a lifestyle that builds upon itself. The quality and alignment of the functional movements you practice is of the utmost importance in order to prevent injury, to improve posture, and to enhance performance in all activities and in life. Functional training is not about going to extremes but rather about consistently participating in a practice that frames a foundation for everything else. It is conditioning for life. Fitness studios with a functional philosophy, such as Alkalign, help train your brain and your body *simultaneously* so that each part is equally strengthened, lengthened, stretched, and mobilized. Functional movement in the way we practice it at Alkalign is the proprietary application of years of research to ensure our clients can experience the immediate benefits of exercise and also invest in their long-term health and reduce overall risk. It's also why we focus not only on functional movement, but also on functional nutrition with a program called Nourish.

In other words, understanding and appreciating a functional approach to life is like learning about your first car. I remember the first time I contributed to the upkeep of my 1983 Volkswagen Rabbit in high school. It was a hunk of junk, but I washed it, vacuumed it, and treated it well because it was the only car I had. I wanted to take care of it. I wish I had invested as much energy into taking care of my own body back then instead of stuffing it with Snackwell's and Skittles. I treated my car better than my body. But instead of dwelling on the past, I'm leveraging my missteps to better inform my future and the future of my clients who trust me with helping them take better care of their bodies.

And while I hope that someday functional fitness gets the acknowledgment and universal adoption it deserves, I hope it never becomes a fad because it's too important to be fleeting. A functional approach to fitness and nutrition is the best way to live a full and healthy life because it doesn't have to hurt to work.

CHOOSE PROGRESS OVER PERFECTION

I honestly never thought anything could measure up to running. I certainly didn't think I'd expect to enjoy something else even more, especially something that can't be measured in the same way. But the reality is that sometimes you don't appreciate something until you fear it might be lost. Again.

Although I'm over two decades into my mental and physical transformation, I still get caught off guard. As much as I try to proactively manage my nutrition, I still sometimes feel like I'm playing Russian-gut roulette when I eat out at a restaurant. And as much as I have dedicated my life to providing an alternative to the bullshit fitness myths, I still fall prey to the mental mind games and the perceived pressure to look and be a certain way. Most recently, my ego got caught up in the idea of going for a run. Yes, me, the person who has spent years writing a book about why I don't run. I was on vacation, and "everyone else was doing it." So I did, too. I quite literally slipped on my shoes, because the laces didn't even tie, and off I went. One foot in front of the other. Across the asphalt and as fast as I could go. I felt like Forrest Gump. It felt like old times. I will spare you the details, but it didn't end well. An MRI revealed that my ACL repair from 27 years prior had been compromised, as well as the cartilage in my knee. Once I moved beyond the initial shame and embarrassment that I should "know better," I accepted this as another reminder of how important it is to take care of yourself for the long haul and heed the warning signs along the way. My ego and knee will recover, but if I keep beating myself up over this blunder, my sense of self will never be the same. At the end of the day, we are all human. We are all doing the best we can with what we've got. That path to self-acceptance isn't easy, but it sure beats the alternative.

The reality is that we are all a work in progress, and progress is, hands down, a healthier mindset than perfection. As much as I wish I could, I can't go back and change the past, and neither can you. All we can do is look at what is and decide if that is what we want going forward. For me, I let those moments teach me about making better choices in the present and in the future. And better choices for me are functional fitness and functional nutrition. A holistic, integrative approach to whole body health and wellness that serves me well today and will do so for decades to come.

My Challenge to You: Whatever your challenges, obstacles, or excuses to doing the best with what you've got and living a more integrated, functional way of life, nothing is ultimately more important than your health. You can wait until something goes awry, or you can proactively invest in the most precious asset you will ever have: *you*. This looks like functional exercise movement, nutrient-rich food, quality sleep, and authentic human connection. Rather than tackling it all at once, pick one thing, and dedicate an hour to it each day this week. One hour is 4% of your day. Your health is 100% of your being. Without it, there is no work or play, no family obligations or amazing vacations.

The question is, *are you willing to invest 4% of your day to move toward a more functional lifestyle? If so, what one small thing will you focus on changing or improving today?* Grab your journal or your notes app, and write it down. Then go do it.

CONCLUSION:
IT DOESN'T
HAVE TO HURT
TO WORK

"Nothing is absolute. Everything changes, everything moves, everything revolves, everything flies and goes away."

Frida Kahlo

Hear me out when I say this book isn't just about fitness or nutrition. It's about *living*, and not just the "breathing and going through the motions" kind of existence. I'm talking about the "jump out of bed because you can't wait to start your day" kind of living. The kind of life where you feel well mentally, physically, and emotionally. The kind of life where you have energy to move your body, to think clearly, to live without aches, pains, and other conditions that impede your ability to enjoy life on a daily basis. The kind of life where you can stop punishing yourself for everything you aren't and accept everything you are. The kind of life where you can be the best version of you. The kind of life where you can nourish your body and *thrive*.

Although I do not and never will proclaim to have all the answers, I do hope that sharing my journey of finding a healthy, functional way of life sparks something in you. Maybe a small seed has been planted that will flourish and grow over time as it did for me. Maybe looking back and understanding where some of your deeply rooted beliefs about your body, food, fitness, and your mindset regarding achievement come from will allow you to accept and work with them versus being controlled by them. Maybe you'll be inspired to look at the way you live your life through a different, more holistic lens. Maybe you'll learn to be a little less hard on yourself for not living up to the unrealistic expectations placed on you by yourself, by others, and by this airbrushed world we live in.

And my ultimate hope for you is that you realize *your body doesn't have to hurt to work.* You can start today to prioritize rather than punish yourself when it comes to your workouts, your diet and food plans, your summer swimsuit choices, and your overall health. Believe me, your future self will thank you. Rather than looking good to look good, I believe we feel good to look good. When you feel better about the way you move and nourish your body, you will feel better about the way you look, no matter the size.

Finding my answer to living a functional way of life took me hitting rock bottom physically, doing a deep dive into my own denial, making slow choices in a fast-paced world of food and fitness, and, eventually, starting my own exercise studios. I also went back to wearing one-piece jumpsuits, which was a sign my body was healing from the inside out.

Not all of us will travel the same path, and that's OK. But we can still learn from each other. And if there's anything you learn from me, I hope it's that living a holistic, functional life truly is the best way, for both your physical and mental well-being.

Here are a few more tips I've found helpful for developing a functional mindset when it comes to everyday movement and nourishment of your body.

MOMENTUM ISN'T A MUSCLE

Then it comes to movement and exercise, and a whole slew of other things in life, momentum is certainly helpful, but *it's not a muscle.* Per Newton's first law of motion, an object in motion stays in motion. I tell myself this every time the alarm goes off in the wee hours of the morning, and I have to get up to teach or take a 6 a.m. class. (I also remind myself to shut off the screen and go to bed earlier because sleep is as important as exercise.) On those days when my eyes feel super-glued shut and every part of my bed is beckoning me to stay at rest, I literally *will* myself to "just stand up." *Just stand up, Erin.* Because once I'm up, I'll stay up. Same for you, too. Even a half-asleep human in motion stays in motion. As hard as it is to transition from rest to motion, if you rely on a little bit of momentum to get you going in the morning, it works. If I can persuade myself to "just get up to pee," or "just take a minute to brush your teeth," then I'm usually good to go to stay in motion for the rest of the morning. The initial obstacle is the hardest. Once I'm up, inertia overcomes exhaustion, and I'm on my way, always grateful for a productive, albeit early, start to the day. But when it comes to the actual exercises themselves, this is not the momentum I'm referring to.

I am not an expert in momentum, or in physics for that matter. In fact, I think physics might have been my lowest grade in high school (something that was initially hard for this overachiever to admit). However, when it comes to movement, exercise, and "working out," I have witnessed the dangers and diminishing returns of momentum. When I see folks in a traditional gym lifting as much as they possibly can and then watch as the weights come crashing down in a thunderous roar in front of them, I shake my head and think unkind thoughts, like *you idiot*. First, because it's dangerous and you could break a foot or injure someone around you. Second, you're missing the benefit of half the workout. To *lift* is one thing. To *lower* is something entirely different. Lifting and lowering both require work to execute correctly and effectively. Letting gravity and momentum take over is a passive, and potentially perilous, alternative.

Take biceps curls as an example. As you bend the elbow and "curl" the weight toward you, the biceps shortens in a *concentric* contraction. When you straighten the arm, you lengthen the biceps in an *eccentric* contraction. It takes more strength to work with gravity and control momentum on the way down than it does to work against gravity on the way up. That's why eccentric muscle work is showing up in more rehabilitation and clinical centers.[25] Incorporating eccentric training increases muscle, boosts metabolism, improves flexibility and performance, and reduces risk of injury. It improves your body's function mechanically and physiologically. Fascinating! Thus, letting gravity take over on the way down deprives you of more than half of your opportunity to build strength, not to mention the wear and tear it causes to your joints.

Along the same lines as momentum are the concepts of acceleration and deceleration. I often observe people using momentum to accelerate their body toward or away from gravity. Here's what I mean: Next time you're at the gym, in a fitness class, or checking out workout videos online, watch how fast individuals move when they lengthen their arms during biceps curls, lower their body during push-ups, or move in the downward direction during lunges. Acceleration in the direction of the ground is the result of the passive pull of gravity and is not representative of one's strength. Acceleration away from gravity using momentum, as in the example of a kipping pull-up or an unintentional hip thrust at the top of a squat or burpee, is also not representative of muscular strength. Both can result in excessive load to the joints, and the risk increases further when you add load and/or speed. Acceleration happens when you use momentum as a muscle, which it's not. It is also the reason I see a lot of snapping of the elbows as the arms lengthen in biceps curls or pull-ups. To me, this is absolutely cringeworthy for two reasons. First and foremost, it's an injury waiting to happen. And second, it's a waste of time and energy. It's much more effective, not to mention safer, to make the most of your movement by going slowly and decelerating on the downward motion toward gravity versus letting gravity steal your workout with a fast snap. That's why you will never see us practice exercises in our studios that use terms such as *clean, jerk,* or *snatch*. Ouch. They all sound like they hurt. In theory, I understand that training your body at a much higher level will prepare you for the mundane moments in life. Sure, snatching 700 pounds from the ground makes taking out the trash a simple task and benching 3 times your body weight makes putting that box of holiday decorations on the top shelf a breeze. It also introduces *a ton* of potential risk, especially since most people are never taught how to move properly while doing that kind of heavy lifting.

Having the mental and physical wherewithal to leverage your strength to align, stabilize, and move well is challenging enough with just your body weight. Being able to do it consistently while also adding weight and acceleration makes the mission nearly impossible. This explains why so many people end up injured. Of course, these injuries are not limited to Olympic weightlifters and CrossFit clients. Whether you're in a physically demanding profession, like first responders, military members, movers, and delivery drivers, or you are a weekend warrior who spends Monday through Friday sitting at your desk, learning to move properly and with control, both mental and muscular, is important.

For the average person like you and me, I believe adding excessive weight to a workout is unnecessary, especially when it is not accompanied by the mind–body connection required to execute safely. What's more important for us is alignment and stability. That's why one of our key phrases at Alkalign is *momentum isn't a muscle*, at least not one that we want to exercise in our practice. Our workouts are designed to give our participants all of the reward with none of the risk because we focus on mindful movement that is balanced in all the right ways. We believe proper movement and alignment help people live better lives by improving strength, enhancing performance, and reducing the risk of injury. And encouraging clients to slow down and focus on control versus the gravitational pull of movementum is a big part of the education. So back to where this section began: *eccentric training*. Eccentric training isn't absolutely everything, but it is a big part of a balanced approach to functional fitness where you can focus your momentum on your movement rather than use it like a muscle.

MEASUREMENT DOES NOT MATTER

Long ago, before the days of fitness apps and trackers, in a land without smartphones or Siri, there were Excel spreadsheets, *and I loved them*. Part of it was my finance profession; the other part was my super-charged, type-A personality. By day, I lived in a world of financial models and revenue projections. By night, I meticulously tracked every metric of my seven to ten workouts per week, believing that I'd lose weight and perform better if my calories out exceeded my calories in. Cardio consumed me. I recorded the length, time, and pace of every swim, run, and bike ride. I monitored average, high, and median heart rate, as well as calories burned. Every. Single. Day. This went on until the morning I woke up and realized I wasn't having fun anymore (that and the hip replacement warning). Excessive training and obsessive tracking were proving exhausting. The constant focus on external metrics and the search for extrinsic validation were making me miserable. So I stopped. Cold turkey (or at least if felt like cold turkey at the time). No more heart rate monitors. No more spreadsheets. No more overanalyzing every meal. And here's what happened when I stopped tracking my workouts:

I started tuning in. Instead of obsessing about what the heart rate monitor said, I listened to my body. Instead of paying attention to my watch, I paid attention to my form. Instead of believing that my workout was a time to "check out," I took advantage of the opportunity to pay attention and to be present in mind and body.

I exercised less and ate better. I stopped over-exercising and replaced intense workouts with more strength- and stretching-based exercises. I took days off from working out and embraced things like mobility and meditation, which challenged me on a whole new level. Less output helped me curb carb cravings and fuel my body with healthy fats and protein versus sugar.

I lost weight and gained strength. I used to believe that if I wasn't burning 1,000 calories per hour and sweating profusely, a workout wasn't legitimate. When I stopped obsessing about the data, I started eating and exercising intuitively. I cut the cardio in favor of strengthening practices that increased muscle and revved my metabolism. The result: unexpected weight loss.

I was less stressed. I didn't realize it at the time, but the constant feeling that I had to achieve something quantitative was stressful. Even when I wasn't competing in a race, I was competing with myself. A number on the scale or the readout of a monitor could make or break my day, a reaction so deeply ingrained but so counterproductive to my wellness. Once I stopped tracking, I stopped worrying.

I realized that the metrics don't paint the whole picture. Metrics aren't always as objective as we think. Just as a scale at the doctor's office needs to be calibrated, so do machines and trackers. Readings can vary, as can what's recorded. Your heart rate reading can be influenced by your hydration, sleep, or how well you've recovered from a previous workout. The metrics aren't fixed, which means relying on them as your sole source of information (and validation) doesn't always give you an accurate snapshot of your workouts.

I had more fun. My relationship with exercise completely changed. It shifted from something I *had* to do to something I *get* to do. It went from punishment to privilege as it became one of my top priorities and more enjoyable on all levels.

I was more honest with myself. Of course, this transformation wasn't always easy, and the shift in mindset was hard at times. During the process of shedding my tracking obsession, I experienced waves of guilt, anxiety, and data-addiction detox. It was hard to put down the watch. I had a looming feeling that if a workout wasn't recorded, it didn't happen. My transformation from being *imprisoned* by my food and fitness choices to feeling *empowered* by these areas of my life happened slowly over time. Gradually, there were glimpses of change. I noticed that I could go for a run and still feel great even if I didn't measure the time, distance, or speed. I recognized that the world continued to turn even when I forgot to record a workout. And somewhere along the way, I broke free of the self-imposed expectations and have never looked back.

Ultimately, this process taught me that information is important—but what we do with it is even more important. Whether you choose to use every gadget available or you like to keep your workouts analog and simple, be sure to check in with how you feel. This is the greatest (and often the only) measurement you need. Your worth is more than a number on a scale, dashboard, or spreadsheet. And often, ignoring those numbers might be the key to greater health and happiness. Measurement does NOT matter when it comes to proving your worth today or investing in your long-term health for the future.

WALK BEFORE YOU RUN

Walking is arguably the functional movement we do most in life but, ironically, the one we never focus on learning. Unless there are extenuating circumstances, we completely take for granted that we can, and always will be able to, walk. We don't think about how alignment and form impact our walking until something goes wrong and we are forced to relearn what was already rooted. This may sound silly since we all move and walk around all day, but in general, innate movements are not something we learned how to do *properly*. We just do them. As infants, we learned to roll over, crawl, sit, and pull up to standing. Eventually we combined standing with the form of walking. Shortly after walking came running. But if doing these movements is part of our primal progression of growing up, how do we know if we're doing them properly? Who taught you how to walk, run, sit, or rotate? Chances are you got up one day when you were a toddler and started walking, accompanied by the celebratory cheers of your small circle of loved ones. Unless you had an extenuating circumstance, you were likely not sent to walking school. Rather, you learned everything about your gait and your posture from those around you.

The same is true for all types of movement, including the seven functional movements. We do them by necessity without ever learning the proper mechanics of how to squat, lunge, hinge, or walk. Yet functional movements are the building blocks to more compound movements. The best next step for all of us (no pun intended) is to go back to the basics of functional movement. *Walking* is the gateway to running, skipping, and skiing. *Lunging* is the starting point for climbing stairs. *Pushing* and *pulling* are the prequel to so many things, including opening doors and operating lawn mowers and shopping carts. Each functional movement is the foundation for another layer of movement. Much like the foundation of a house, if the integrity of even one functional movement is compromised, the entire structure is negatively impacted. But if the foundation is firm and built well using basic but crucial building principles, then your structure is secure even when there are a few storms.

When I started running cross country and track, I was given workouts to help me run faster so I could be more competitive. The name of the game was to win, to cross the finish line first or as close to that as possible. Faster was better. The *fartlek* (a Swedish word meaning "speed play") was essential to training. Form was not a concern unless it got in the way of speed. I was pretty fast, so my form was never identified as an issue. As much as I wish someone had educated me on alignment and its connection to performance and injury prevention back then, I'm pretty sure it would not have resonated anyway. Developmentally, the brain of the tween, teen, and 20-year-old is different at each stage. Young bodies are resilient. And our young minds convince us that we wear a cloak of invincibility. We take a hard fall and get right back up. But our ability to rebound and recover changes over time. It hurts more to fall as we get older, and it takes longer to get up. We bounce back at a slower pace, or sometimes not at all. I'm guessing I can skip the examples here because most of you are probably nodding your head and remembering the last time you had a hard time recovering from something you used to consider "small."

What I also failed to realize for my first three decades on Earth is that the body is very smart and adapts quickly. Oftentimes, it will do what it needs to do to get the job done, even if that path from A to B is not the best. I got where I needed to go, despite crooked hips, pronating feet, misaligned knees, and virtually zero gluteal or core engagement. Thanks to equal parts mindlessness, momentum, and denial, I was able to put one foot in front of the other. I even ran a sub 3:40 marathon to qualify for the Boston Marathon. But my point-in-time performance was not indicative of future permanence. I didn't think about how running with my left hip leading my body would throw off my alignment. I didn't understand the connection between poor form and the pain it would later cause or how my high number of miles run per week was expediting the wear and tear on my body. I wrongly assumed that what was would always be. I failed to recognize the biological tax running was applying to my body because I never really learned how to properly walk *or* run.

Nailing the fundamentals such as learning to walk properly before learning to run properly is crucial for progress, performance, and preservation. At Alkalign, we teach the basics first and layer on from there. This progression is what we refer to as *align, stabilize, and move.* We prioritize alignment in order to protect the joints. We continually practice mindful movement in a controlled environment with a lot of coaching and feedback because our goal is to establish healthy movement habits that will translate into everyday tasks and activities. And we do this together as a community, in a welcoming and supportive environment where everyone is willing to be held accountable. Together, we learn how to *walk before we run.*

TOMORROW STARTS TODAY

With years of life coaching, business coaching, and an abundance of self-help books, I have had the opportunity to reflect in my own mirror. At this point, it's obvious just how ego-driven I was in my younger years, always caring about grades, class rank, race-podium placement, run times, calories burned, medals hanging on my wall, clothing sizes and labels, and so on. It's not surprising given that I grew up in what I affectionately refer to as a "quantitative environment." My father in particular placed a lot of well-intentioned emphasis on things that could be measured. The easiest topics to engage in conversationally were always related to my GPA, salary, or marathon times. I don't ever remember talking about whether I was enjoying my studies or feeling fulfilled in my work. This was neither good nor bad. It was simply what I knew.

When I was doing all that soul searching in my 20s and 30s, I came to realize I loved teaching fitness, paying attention to movement, and learning about healthy bodies, healthy nutrition, and healthy minds. But most of all, I loved connecting with people. I loved the exchange of information in conversation and the ability to both teach and learn from each other all at the same time. I realized I didn't necessarily care about climbing the corporate ladder and making the top salary. I realized I was willing to piss off my ego for the sake of following my soul and pursuing my purpose. And thus, the first big shift in my life started to take place. That's when Coach Mary challenged me to look in my proverbial mirror. She encouraged me to challenge my assumptions by asking, *is it true?* And she encouraged me to realize that tomorrow starts today.

The choices you and I make today affect how we live our lives tomorrow. And how we view tomorrow affects how we live today. Let that sink in for a few moments.

In fact, my favorite entrepreneurial inspiration comes from a daily blog by author and entrepreneur Seth Godin. It's the first thing I read every morning. And one day this message appeared in my inbox:

> "Perhaps it's time to do something else. Not a new job, or a new city, but perhaps a different story. A story about possibility and sufficiency. A story about connection and trust. A story about *for* and *with*, instead of *at* or *to*. Bootstrapping your way to a new story about the world around you is one of the most difficult things you'll ever do. Our current story was built piecemeal, over time, the result of vivid interactions and hard-fought lessons. But if that story isn't getting you where you need to go, then what's it for? It's entirely possible that the story we tell ourselves all day every day is true and accurate and useful, the very best representation of the world as it actually is. It's possible, but vanishingly unlikely. What if we search for a useful story instead?"

So what kind of useful story are we going to live tomorrow that starts today? Your health is your lifestyle. Whether you smoke cigarettes and eat Twinkies or exercise and sip green juice, your health is something that impacts your daily decisions. And over time, as we make healthier choices, we evolve into a seasoned version of ourselves. Every day, we have the opportunity to learn and grow, and when we know better, we can do better. It's not about walking the tightrope to perfection. It's not about living the extremes where it has to work to hurt. It's about simply learning how to walk properly, finding a dynamic balance in our lives, and realizing tomorrow starts today.

FINDING MY ANSWER IN ALKALIGN

Learning and realizing over time that our bodies didn't have to hurt to work meant finding a tangible answer for my desire to consistently live a functional way of life. And Alkalign was my answer.

After six years of owning my studios as a franchisee, I was ready for something more in 2015. I was living in an ego-dominant industry and operating under an ego-driven brand, and I was tired of selling the bikini-body aesthetics of the "long and lean" exterior with no focus on the interior. I now had two precious daughters who were watching, observing, and learning from my every move. That's when Coach Mary challenged me to look in the metaphorical mirror of my life, which was an often-uncomfortable experience yet one that resulted in incredible clarity. I could no longer deny the perfectionist tendencies I suffered from for much of my life. And I woke up one day during my time with Coach Mary and realized that the unrealistic expectations were making me miserable. I'll be the first to admit there is nothing perfect about misery. Slowly, over time, I eased up on the pursuit of perfection, the measuring and the judging. I was tired of feeling shame and assigning blame when something didn't go right. And, quite frankly, I was tired of caring what other people thought. Instead of worrying about the fallout from things like not showing up to my work retreat because I was in the middle of a painful miscarriage, I invested in myself and the things that mattered: my family, my friends, my business, my health, and myself. I finally learned to check my ego at the door and embrace what *was* in the present moment. I conceived Alkalign with a mission in mind—it was developed with a higher purpose for people with a higher purpose.

But Alkalign didn't happen immediately. It took a lot of thoughtful preparation and planning to turn my barre-based studios into functional movement studios of my own. Rather than react to what wasn't right at a surface level, I took the time to understand "the why" behind the biomechanics of the body in order to create an alternative that was both physically and psychologically sustainable. In fact, Alkalign Studios is in many ways a by-product of one of my other careers as a Six Sigma project manager. Six Sigma is a disciplined, data-driven methodology for eliminating defects in a system. It aims to find and address the *root cause* in order to eliminate further issues, errors, and defects rather than the alternate and often temporary "Band-Aid" solution. When I decided to pivot from my niche barre studio to a more holistic, functional fitness offering, I first identified everything that wasn't working, aka the defects. From the exercise movements to the messages we were sending our clients and our team, we systematically evaluated and eliminated anything that would potentially cause harm to our body and our sense of self. This meant we removed traditional barre movements like "tucking" and "marching," as well as exercises like "round back on the wall" or "round back chair" as we felt that the potential risk of these exercises was greater than the potential reward. We replaced Jimmy Choo shoe cues and promises of bikini bodies with anatomical information and functional education on everyday movements for everyday people. We shifted our messaging from the external to the internal, from the extrinsic to the intrinsic, from exclusive to inclusive. The goal was to provide all of the good and none of the bad—all of the soul without the ego. Our focus was on the rewards of a mindful, sustainable, and effective movement practice while reducing, if not eliminating, the risk of injury. And we kept telling ourselves and our clients that *it doesn't have to hurt to work.*

On the outside, Alkalign is a fitness studio. On the inside, it's so much more. Movement education is at the heart of what we do. Community is at the heart of who we are. And a comprehensive, challenging, and very effective workout with immediate benefits is what we deliver. It is proven. Time and time again, Alkalign is the place that helps people feel better. It's the place they return to when they are beaten up and broken down from everything else. It provides all of the reward of exercise without any of the risks that many other types of fitness or misinformed ways of viewing nutrition present.

And Alkalign works because it is designed with you—the whole you—in mind. We offer a holistic, customized approach to fitness, everyday movements, and nutrition. And we're focused on safety, sustainability, and the long-term physical and mental health of clients. This comes in the form of strength, flexibility, mobility, balance, proprioception, and, perhaps most of all, *authentic human connection*. No gimmicks. No fancy equipment. No diets. No bullshit or airbrushed portrayals of what we "should" be. It's all about you and your relationship to your goals and your center of gravity. The "lack of flash" at Alkalign doesn't detract from our ability to be innovative, effective, and fun. The real power is in the simplicity of our practice.

Over the past 12-plus years, six years as a barre studio franchisee and six years as the owner and CEO of Alkalign, I have taught thousands of alignment-based fitness classes and have worked with tens of thousands of people. Due to the inclusive and safe nature of Alkalign exercises, we attract a diverse clientele compared to other forms of fitness. Which means I've had the opportunity to study real bodies in real time on a daily basis. And it's the consistency of these encounters that inspires me as I pay attention to my clients' alignment, to their form, even to the look on their faces when they're in our classes. My clients know I give a shit about them, not just about what's happening anatomically, but what's happening on the inside and how that impacts everything else in their lives, too. I see the whole picture of who they really are, and I have a desire to understand what it's like to be in their shoes. Each conversation, no matter how small or fleeting, is enjoyable and informational. Each connection is an investment. And each interaction is an opportunity to help people help themselves. This philosophy and desire to help people know themselves and heal themselves is reflected in the company and culture of Alkalign. Alkalign is a brand, a practice, and a community our clients can trust.

But I recognize that Alkalign isn't for everyone. There are other workouts making people feel stronger and healthier every day. However, my goal with Alkalign has never been, and will never be, to be the biggest company or fitness brand. It's to be the *most trusted*. And we educate and empower you so you trust yourself. That's what makes us successful in more ways than one.

Alkalign has been my answer because I created it with a specific goal in mind. I wanted a workout that would include everything I needed and nothing that I didn't. I had tried every workout known to man (and woman) and could never find one that had all the elements. So I decided to develop something that included a balanced approach to strength, mobility, and low-impact cardio with an emphasis on the education and execution. To move is one thing. To move well is something totally different. We optimize the functional movements that really matter by prioritizing quality over quantity, and we do the same with Nourish, our nutrition program. We also refuse to accept busyness as a badge and encourage a mindful approach in all areas of life. And these same principles apply to our business operations, relationships, parenting, community engagement, and pretty much everything else in life. That's why Alkalign isn't just *my* answer; it's been the answer for hundreds of others, too.

THE BLUE CREW

People ask me all the time what my "target market" is when it comes to my fitness studios. Investors, potential franchisees, and curious clients are all looking for the very specific type of person who can be easily targeted on social media using a simple formula such as "women ages 25-45 with an interest in Lululemon, tennis, and rosé all day." But Alkalign doesn't work that way. It's not a demographic. It's a psychographic. *It's a group of people who share a mindset around health and wellness.* It is people who are invested in their health for the long term. They give a shit about more than how a workout immediately impacts their waistline. They think critically and are curious about the way their bodies work; they want to learn about the best movements and food choices for their particular bodies; and they want to protect and preserve their health as an investment for their future. My clients want to do the best with what they've got. And my team is trained and equipped to help them do just that.

Due to our proximity to Stanford University, we attract a large population of doctors and health professionals to our classes. We also have clients who are teenagers, octogenarians, and every age in between. There are men and women of all different shapes, sizes, and colors. But the one thing they all have in common is a high commitment to their best selves. At Alkalign, *we seek to educate, empower, and inspire clients to know better so they can do better.* Clients appreciate the level of sophistication we offer, and they're thirsty for the knowledge and empowerment that comes from understanding which muscle they're working at any given time and how functional movement impacts physical, mental, and emotional health.

I have veteran clients who have trained with me for years leveraging the foundation they build in our studios to continue to do all the other things they love: tennis, golf, soccer, cycling, running, horseback riding, and skiing. And I love to see new clients overcome physical and emotional pain that has been with them for decades. Our proprietary workout combination of strength, flexibility, balance, mobility, and mindset prepare them for life not only physically, but also mentally and emotionally. And I watch with joy and pride the correlation between the strength they build in their bodies and the resilience they build in their minds as they navigate the ups and downs of life because of the foundation they have in place while at Alkalign. Never was this more true than during the COVID-19 crisis.

As our world turned upside down in 2020, we pivoted our instruction format in a matter of 24 hours and came up with an online-only offering. The Blue Crew put on their growth mindset hats and got to work. They signed up and showed up, side-planking from their living rooms on the other side of the screen. They squeezed in the self-care whenever they could between tending to patients at the hospital, managing teams online, and putting out fires on the home front. I attribute their ability to respond versus react, to support versus slam, and to connect versus criticize to the inherently amazing humans they are and the skills they have honed while a part of our program. While we may have all been carrying heavier emotional and mental loads during the pandemic, we were mindful of not physically carrying the pain, as long as we didn't have to. I'm so proud of the Blue Crew and their commitment to a functional way of life, no matter the circumstances. Because when you know better, you do better.

DEAR FUTURE YOU

As you can tell, I am ridiculously passionate about what I practice and what I preach, which are nowadays one in the same: *a functional approach to life*. But if you've made it this far with me, you know as well as I do that it wasn't always that way. It took a long time for me to break free from my deeply rooted beliefs about fitness and nutrition before I could even consider another perspective or adopt a different way of doing things. I had to acknowledge the disconnect between how I saw my current self and my future self. Believe it or not, this disconnect is no joke.

Research out of UCLA and Stanford has indicated a psychological disconnect between the current and the future self for most of us. We think of our future selves as different people, which could explain why many of us don't connect the dots between how current lifestyle choices can impact future health and wellness.

UCLA social psychologist and assistant marketing professor Hal Hershfield studies these ideas. In 2015, a UCLA news release about Hershfield's work explained his findings this way: "While we routinely make sacrifices for the people we feel closest to—our spouses, children, and parents—and will even give money or our time to help complete strangers, like the homeless, the one person whose plight we may actually ignore is our future self." Hershfield said in the release that people thinking of themselves in the future see a different person, a stranger.[26]

The news release also explains that Hershfield has "found that the emotional disconnect we have with the person we will become in 20 to

40 years could explain, for example, why many people don't save enough for retirement; why they continue to indulge in unhealthy behaviors, accepting the risk of incurring terrible diseases in the future; and why they make bad ethical decisions despite knowing that they might suffer consequences down the road."

To arrive at these conclusions, researchers used fMRI technology to observe neural patterns when subjects thought about their future selves. The researchers observed that these patterns "were most similar to the neural patterns that arose when thinking about another person. In other words, on a brain level, the future self 'looked' like another person."[27]

Making the connection between our current selves and our future selves is crucial for making healthy, functional decisions today. Remember, tomorrow starts today. And this connection requires alignment between who we are, who we want to be tomorrow, and who we want to be 20 years from now. Which means alignment isn't just for our bodies, it's for our lives.

ALIGNMENT MATTERS

During past seasons of my life, I desperately wanted to believe that exercise is "all you need." I wanted to believe that my studios were the answer to everyone's questions, the solution to all problems. Truth is, there is more to the equation. From our physical well-being to the social and emotional parts of us, there are many dials that need to be in balance for us to live our best selves. But I know that aligning your food and fitness goals and matching them with your mindset is key to moving forward.

Alkalign Studios, in person or online, might not be your answer to alignment, and that's OK. But understanding body alignment is the foundation for movement for your life. Learning about nutrition principles is key to nourishing your body from the inside out. The two go together and also have to be aligned with all of the other inputs you balance from day to day. Too much of a good thing isn't good if that input is grossly out of alignment. And once something in your life is grossly out of alignment, your body will tell you. Remember: it doesn't have to hurt to work. So, *live present, be forward, and find your way back to making your life functional in every area—your fitness, your food, and your mindset. This is my ultimate challenge to you.*

EPILOGUE:
IT'S YOUR TURN

"You only live once, but if you do
it right, once is enough."

Mae West

At the end of the day, we are all a work in progress when it comes to living holistic, functional lifestyles. So start where you are, with your current self. Here's how:

Set a goal for where you want your future self to end up.

Establish SMART (specific, measurable, attainable, relevant, time-based) goals to get there. Prepare for the barriers that will stand in your way.

Be flexible and resilient.

Stay the course.

Realize you're capable of accomplishing anything you want to.

Commit to getting out of your own way.

Don't let perfection be the enemy of progress, (or as Ava told me at age 8, "Practice makes better, Mommy, not perfect.")

Don't be afraid to order off-menu.

And remember, *it doesn't have to hurt to work.*

EPILOGUE PART TWO:
THE ALKALIGN EPILOGUE

A common question we hear is, "What does Alkalign mean?" We took the word *alkaline*, which represents water, stability, and balance and also refers to the ideal pH state of your body, and combined it with our passion for alignment to form *Alkalign*.

And here is our manifesto:

At Alkalign, we embrace what is real, raw, and human.
We infuse principles of strength, alignment, and
nourishment to surface our ultimate selves.
We are a team of individuals, a family of originals.
We are grounded, we are charged.

We believe that balance is dynamic and doesn't
always mean staying in the middle.
We dare to step outside of our comfort zones because
we have a foundation of strength to return to.
We practice what is proven but believe forward motion brings stability.

Live present. Be forward.
Alkalign

Alkalign is training for life. Our functional fitness classes train your body and your brain to work together to prepare them for everyday tasks. Whether you are squatting to pick up a heavy box or rotating to grab something from the back seat, our proprietary blend of exercises ensures that your entire body is strong, balanced, and mobile so that you live well and without pain. Alkalign is more than a workout. In addition to high-quality and effective group fitness classes, we offer a holistic approach to health and wellness.

RESOURCES:
A FEW OF MY FAVORITES

To say I'm fascinated with biomechanics and a functional way of life is an understatement. I have spent nearly half of my life studying the way the human body works. Here are my top three resources I return to on a weekly, sometimes daily, basis:

Move Your DNA by biomechanist Katy Bowman
Whole Body Barefoot by Katy Bowman
The Roll Model by Yoga Tune Up founder Jill Miller, the rolling, mobility, and blue-ball queen

ACKNOWLEDGEMENTS:
MY DREAM TEAM

"Feeling gratitude and not expressing it is like wrapping a present and not giving it."

William Arthur Ward

I want to thank my "dream team" for everything you have contributed to my life. I have the most incredible friends, family, and Blue Crew. It takes a village, and I am grateful you are part of mine:

Tony, my husband, partner in all things business and life, and Mr. Alkalign himself. You have been unwavering in your support since the very beginning. Thank you for allowing me the space to create and always offering encouragement to pursue one outlandish idea after another.

Lizzie, work wife, little spoon, ginger spice, and COO. I don't know where I'd be without you. I'm not sure how I got so lucky, but I'm grateful every day that you are part of my life. I wouldn't want to be swimming upstream on a mission to disrupt such a messed up industry without you. Thank you for your patience, especially when I'm running late or long.

Mom and *Dad.* I feel incredibly blessed to have been raised in a loving home that provided a foundation for me to continue to grow as an individual, wife, mom, friend, and entrepreneur. I have learned so much from each of you that has helped shape who I am today. I now appreciate how challenging parenting is and am grateful for the investment you made in me with your whole heart and soul.

Ryan, Carey, and *Andrew.* From the womb to the "real world," we've been through so much together. I'm grateful for the shared experiences that will forever bond us. Through road trips in the "way back" and running the Chicago marathon together, you were my first friends and will forever be my favorite people. Special shout-out to the amazing additions to our sibling squad, Noah and Pooky. I'm grateful for your support and generosity and for your agreements to purchase at least one copy of this book each. You are the best.

Bennett, Dylan, and *Quinn.* Although you are technically my nieces, you will always be my three bonus daughters. I love you more than you know and am in awe of your strength, creativity, resilience, and confidence. You have already taught me so much, and I suspect this trend will continue for decades to come. I love that our family is full of girl power, and I promise to do my part to ensure that Team WinSki leaves a positive mark on this world.

Dana W., my first California friend and my ride or die to this day. Your sense of humor alone got me through some pretty dark times. I've never met anyone so accepting no matter what the circumstances. I love that I can call you anytime and you will be there to listen, laugh, and authentically share in life without judgement. Thanks for your support through all the ups and downs of life.

Beth G., my friend and sounding board since 1996. I'm so grateful our paths crossed and continue to intersect in the most timely and profound ways. There is no one I'd rather collaborate on this project with than you. Thank you for your infinite patience and insightful advice. You are truly a gem.

Marlene. Your design creativity and positive attitude are as inspiring as your green thumb. Your ability to take an idea from inception to

Photoshop is amazing. Thank you for being a loyal teammate and friend and for always making me laugh, especially in the most challenging seasons.

Marijane (aka MJ), my friend, fellow Virgo, birthday twin, and editor extraordinaire. You wear many hats in my life, and I'm grateful for your ability to navigate so seamlessly from one to the next. Thank you for always believing in Alkalign and in me. I am truly grateful for the energy you have dedicated to this project. I hope there are many more opportunities to collaborate in our future.

Cathy P., my friend, podcast partner, parenting coach, and, at time of publishing, the most "senior" instructor in Alkalign history. Your wisdom is as abundant as your energy. Thank you for always being there, including the future frantic calls I will be making for advice on raising teenage girls. I can only hope mine turn out as kind, confident and loving of their mama as yours did.

Coach Mary. You have changed my life for the better. I was wounded and confused when I met you. I had no idea which way I was headed, and you helped guide the way to a meaning and a mission that has never been clearer. Thank you for inspiring me to "do the work" and challenging me to push past the obstacles along the way.

Krista, Dan, Matt, and *Katie,* the humans who helped me personify Alkalign. People come into your life for different reasons. You have forever transformed mine, and for that, I thank you.

The beloved Blue Crew. You've stood by through thick and thin. Without you, my mission would not have come to fruition. You show up every day and in every way. Special thanks to everyone who read one of the many iterations of this book—typos and nonsensical segues included. I am equally grateful for the feedback and affirmations you have gifted me along the way.

The amazing Alkalign team of instructors. You have risen to the occasion with every pivot and obstacle along the way. Your commitment to Alkalign and our collective Blue Crew is inspiring. As Helen Keller once said, "Alone we can do so little; together we can do so much."

And last but definitely not least, I want to thank my daughters,

Ava and *Elle.* I didn't know when I started this little parenting adventure that I'd learn as much from you as I hoped to teach in return. I am in awe of the amazing individuals you are becoming. I admire your kindness, confidence, sense of humor, and sense of self. I aspire to be as creative and inquisitive as you are and hope you are as proud of yourselves as I am of you. Love you both to the moon and back × infinity.

NOTES

1. The Lancet, "Over 95% of the world's population has health problems, with over a third having more than five ailments," ScienceDaily, www.sciencedaily.com/releases/2015/06/150608081753.htm.

2. World Health Organization, "Mental health," World Health Organization, https://www.who.int/health-topics/mental-health#tab=tab_2.

3. Dan Siegel, "Mindsight," Mind Your Brain, Inc., https://drdansiegel.com/mindsight/.

4. Justin Sonnenburg and Erica Sonnenburg, *The Good Gut: Taking Control of Your Weight, Your Mood and Your Long-Term Health* (New York: Penguin Press, 2015).

5. Mary M. Yoke and Carol K. Armbruster, *Methods of Group Exercise Instruction* (Champaign, IL: Human Kinetics, 2019), 118.

6. Mayo Clinic Staff, "Functional fitness training: Is it right for you?" Mayo Clinic, Mayo Foundation for Medical Education and Research, September 4, 2019, https://www.mayoclinic.org/healthy-lifestyle/fitness/in-depth/functional-fitness/art-20047680.

7. *Cambridge Advanced Learner's Dictionary & Thesaurus*, 4th ed. (Cambridge: Cambridge University Press, 2013), s.v. "Functional." https://dictionary.cambridge.org/us/dictionary/english/functional.

8. Brené Brown, "Own our history. Change the story," *Brené Brown* (blog), June 18, 2015, https://brenebrown.com/blog/2015/06/18/own-our-history-change-the-story/.

9. Robert Fulghum, *All I Really Need to Know I Learned in Kindergarten: Uncommon Thoughts on Common Things* (New York: Villard Books, 1988).

10. Carol S. Dweck, *Mindset: The New Psychology of Success* (New York: Random House, 2016).

11. Leonard Calabrese, "How mindfulness training can boost your immune system," Health Essentials, Cleveland Clinic, January 15, 2018 https://health.clevelandclinic.org/how-mindfulness-training-can-help-you-achieve-immunologic-health.

12. Matthew Thorpe and Rachael Link, "12 science-based benefits of meditation," Healthline, Healthline Media, last modified October 27, 2020, https://www.healthline.com/nutrition/12-benefits-of-meditation.

13. Maria Cohut, "Mindfulness has 'huge potential' as a weight loss strategy," Medical News Today, Healthline Media UK Ltd., December 30, 2018, https://www.medicalnewstoday.com/articles/324043.

14. "Our definition of a scientist," Science Council, accessed September 1, 2021, https://sciencecouncil.org/about-science/our-definition-of-a-scientist/.

15. Tim Kelley, *True Purpose: 12 Strategies for Discovering the Difference You Are Meant to Make* (Berkeley: Transcendent Solutions Press, 2009).

16. Kelley, *True Purpose*.

17. Scott Barry Kaufman, "The pressing need for everyone to quiet their egos," *Beautiful Minds* (blog), May 21, 2018, https://blogs.scientificamerican.com/beautiful-minds/the-pressing-need-for-everyone-to-quiet-their-egos/#.

18. Anne Craig, "Discovery of 'thought worms' opens window to the mind," *Queen's Gazette* online, July 13, 2020, https://www.queensu.ca/gazette/stories/discovery-thought-worms-opens-window-mind.

19. "Defining critical thinking," Foundation for Critical Thinking, accessed September 3, 2021, https://www.criticalthinking.org/pages/defining-critical-thinking/766.

20. Michael Pollan, *In Defense of Food: An Eater's Manifesto* (New York: Penguin Press, 2008).

21. Mayo Clinic Staff, "Denial: when it helps, when it hurts" Mayo Clinic, Mayo Foundation for Medical Education and Research, April 9, 2020, https://www.mayoclinic.org/healthy-lifestyle/adult-health/in-depth/denial/art-20047926.

22. Philip Hunter, "The inflammation theory of disease: The growing realization that chronic inflammation is crucial in many diseases opens new

avenues for treatment," *EMBO reports* vol. 13,11 (2012): 968-70. doi:10.1038/embor.2012.142.

23. Joshua Rosenthal, "The secret to IIN's health coach program is now scientifically proven," *IIN Blog* (blog), Institute for Integrative Nutrition, Published July 10, 2015; last updated March 4, 2021, https://www.integrativenutrition.com/blog/the-secret-to-iins-health-coach-program-is-now-scientifically-proven.

24. Ann Wigmore, *The Hippocrates Diet and Health Program* (New York: Penguin, 1984), 9.

25. Paul LaStayo et al. "Eccentric exercise in rehabilitation: safety, feasibility, and application," *J Appl Physiol* (1985). 2014 Jun 1;116(11):1426-34. doi: 10.1152/japplphysiol.00008.2013.

26. Cynthia Lee, "The stranger within: connecting with our future selves," UCLA Newsroom online, Regents of University of California, April 9, 2015, https://newsroom.ucla.edu/stories/the-stranger-within-connecting-with-our-future-selves.

27. Lee, "The stranger within."

ABOUT THE AUTHOR

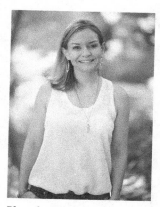

Photo by Nicole Scarborough

Erin J. Paruszewski is a functional fitness enthusiast, holistic health coach, entrepreneur, and the founder and CEO of Alkalign, a health and wellness company that operates boutique functional fitness studios online and in California. Erin's passion is helping others feel better from the inside out. Her innovative and evolving offerings inspire clients to adopt safe, sustainable, and effective lifestyle practices that transform both the body and the mind.